D1246471

YOU WILL ROCK AS A DAD!

THE EXPERT GUIDE TO FIRST-TIME PREGNANCY
AND EVERYTHING NEW FATHERS NEED
TO KNOW

ALEX GRACE

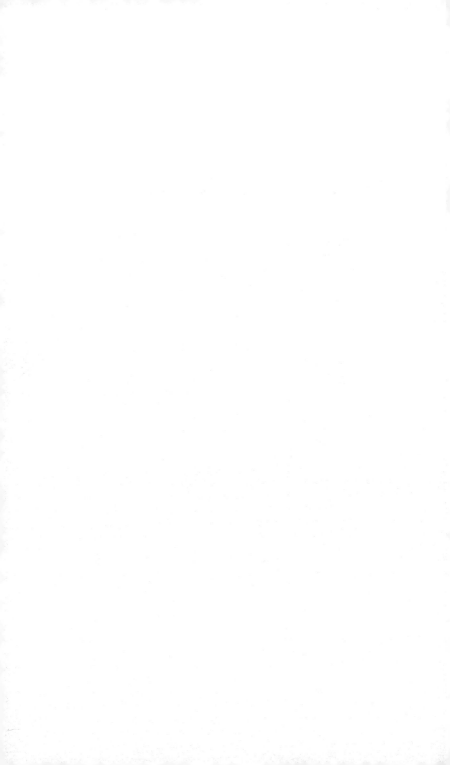

CONTENTS

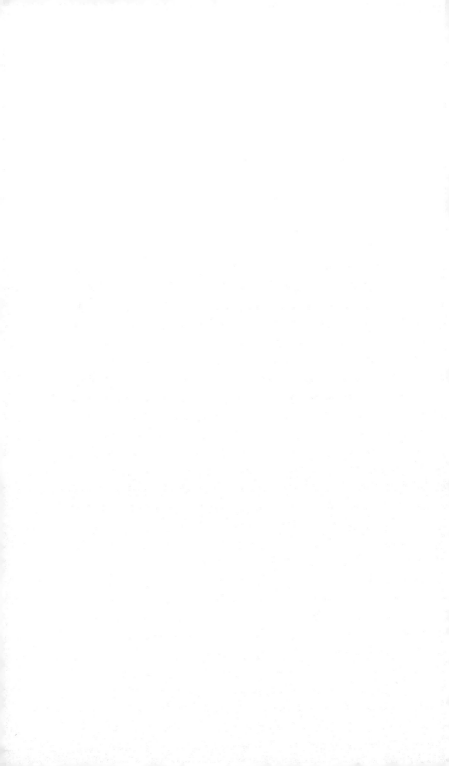

YOU WILL ROCK AS A DAD!

The Expert Guide to First-Time Pregnancy and
Everything New Fathers Need to Know

Alex Grace

indirect, that are incurred as a result of the use of the information contained within this document, including, but not limited to, errors, omissions, or inaccuracies.

❀ Created with Vellum

INTRODUCTION

"The power of a dad in a child's life is
unmatched." —Justin Ricklefs

You've been wanting to be a father ever since you
can remember. You always thought it would happen
one day in the future. When your wife suggested it
was time to start trying to get pregnant, you didn't
hesitate. Most couples sometimes struggle to get
pregnant, so you thought it could take at least a
couple of months. "Trying to get pregnant will be
fun," you thought, and "I'll have the most sex I've had
in my whole life." These thoughts made you feel
excited for the journey ahead.

Until one day, way sooner than you ever thought possible, your wife's waiting for you as you come home after a long day at work. You feel nervous looking at how excited she is. The next minute, she grabs a little white stick and points it so close to your face that you must step back to see what's happening.

You see two blue lines when your eyes eventually focus on the little stick (which now seems like it could be a weapon). What does this even mean? You wonder. Then, suddenly, you realize it might be a sign that your time of sex, whenever you wanted, was over. Carefully choosing your words, you ask, "Does this mean...." Before you can even finish your sentence, your wife shouts, "We're pregnant!"

Suddenly, a wave of emotions hit you. Feelings you can't understand. You always anticipated this to be the happiest day of your life. You have wanted this, so why would you not be ecstatic? But, apart from the apparent feelings of elation, you're suddenly overcome by feelings of extreme fear.

Thoughts are streaming through your head. What if something goes wrong? What if we don't have enough money to raise a child? What if I'm going to be a bad father? I don't know anything about being a dad. What if I can't console my baby when they cry? What if I do something that wrecks my child's life forever? The list of fears and thoughts mull through your head for weeks while you try to put on a brave face. The last thing you want is for your wife to realize that you're petrified at the thought of becoming a father.

If you've nodded in agreement to any of these fears, there's hope. You don't have to go through the next nine months (or the lifetime of being a father after that) alone. You don't have to wonder why your wife is seemingly impossible while pregnant. You don't have to fear the birth process. There's also no reason why you should be afraid of bringing the baby home, bonding with them, or being a good father.

Your fears will soon be a thing of the past. You've come to the right place. You Will Rock As a Dad! will help you through every step of the journey that lies ahead. It'll be the buddy you wish you could ask all the questions over a cold beer but feel too embarrassed to admit these fears to. This book—or buddy, if you will—will never judge you for being scared or asking what you fear might be silly questions.

Instead, this book will give you the support you need during these coming months. It'll help you know what to expect in every step of this pregnancy journey and having a newborn baby to care for. Many dads struggle to connect with their new babies, as they haven't physically carried the baby through pregnancy or given birth. Many dads don't understand the strength of their fatherly instincts, as society tends to focus only on the mother and their instincts in caring for a baby.

Apart from this, you'll need to find a new way of connecting to your wife, as your baby will become her highest priority. Then, you'll also need to find a way to make time for self-care. You'll need to carve time to do things yourself and not just settle into your new routine as a dad.

All of this can be enough to freak many men out, but you don't have to be one of them. There's no need to fear this time. Even though you might feel overwhelmed at times, you'll be ready for them. You Will Rock As a Dad! will also help you to know when your mental health might start to suffer and how to receive support.

About Me

I'm very excited to be helping you along your new journey. As a sports coach, my life is all about teamwork and collaboration. I'm the eldest in a family of five and have always been the fun uncle. But being the go-to family member for your nieces and nephews is nothing like having your own child. Even if you believe you'll be the best dad and love spending time with little ones, the shock of becoming a father can spin your head into such a loop that you might want to work out or do whatever helps blow off some steam and release some cortisol.

Your experience doesn't have to be like this. Helping parents, particularly new dads, find their feet in their new roles is one of my passions. I have a deep love for children, and after working in the childcare system for many years, I understand the attention to detail caring for a child requires. I have experience working with children from many backgrounds, which gives me different perspectives to draw knowledge from. I also have experience in fatherhood, having had the honor of becoming a dad a couple of times and creating my own little sports team at home.

I'm passionate about sharing my knowledge and experience because I know the value this can bring to first-time fathers. So, let's get straight into it and discuss what you should do and know when your wife announces her tummy is about to blow up like a balloon.

1

YOU'RE GOING TO BE A DAD!

You've had enough time to get over the initial shock that your wife's pregnant. At times, you're feeling quite pleased with yourself. After all, this is the best proof ever that your penis does work. Congratulations!

Despite this, you find yourself lying awake at night. You're scared of what lies ahead. Your life is no longer going to revolve around you. Sure, you had to make some adjustments when you got married or entered into a serious relationship with your partner. But, there was always still enough time to go out with the boys or do whatever you felt like. No matter what many people might try to tell you, this is about to change. This is scary. However, the more you educate yourself on the journey that you're embarking on, the less overwhelmed you'll feel.

Having a Child Is Scary

Before we go over the nitty-gritty of pregnancy and caring for a newborn, let's focus on you and what you're likely going through. We've already established two emotions you might be feeling: happiness, maybe more delight and elation, and being so scared that you might even have to run to the toilet more often than usual. Sometimes, you're probably feeling both of those opposing emotions at the same time. Unfortunately for most dads-to-be, the fears of having a pregnant wife often outweigh the happiness or excitement of becoming a father.

You might fear that you're too selfish to be a good dad. Another person's needs will now become more important than your own. You won't be able to be selfish any longer. You'll have to devote hours daily to your family: You'll need to bond with your child, care for this new life, and take care of their mama, whose body will go through absolute hell over these upcoming months. Your time is no longer your own.

Similarly, you'll have to share your money. Having a baby's expensive, and there are just no two ways to avoid that. Diapers alone can break the monthly budget, not to mention all the other things your baby might need, such as formula, creams, medicine, doctor's appointments, clothes, daycare, and so on. Just as your priorities with your time will change, so will your financial responsibilities.

Fortunately, there's a silver lining to this. Many women (especially grandmas and aunts) are attracted to a baby like a magnet. If you need to have a break and have some selfish me-time, give these lovely women in your life a call to ask them to babysit or help your wife. Your wife might even want alone time from you. So do this, or at the very least, discuss this with her.

Like many, a woman's time can seem endless when cooing over a baby, and so can her purse. Have you ever seen a woman in a baby shop? Many tend to go crazy about blowing the budget by buying goodies. If you make sure someone gifts your wife with an oversized baby shower, you'll save a lot of money. Your baby will likely receive so many clothing items or packets of diapers that you might not have to buy as much for your baby as you fear. Make sure to keep the tags on all the clothing items your baby might receive so you can swap them out for different sizes if you need to.

Another fear you might have is loving your job more than your baby. Having this fear is more natural than you might realize. You've been doing your job for many years. You've chosen your career path. You might love your job so much that hours at work can feel like only a couple of minutes. Or maybe you don't like your job all that much. Perhaps you feel like you'll love hanging out with the guys more. This can still apply to you. Now, think back to when you started your first job or when you first met your best friend. Were you not scared of the unknown and failing? Looking back now, those fears seem pretty ridiculous, don't they? The same applies to having your first baby. You don't know what it's like to have your tiny human. You don't realize how you'll be entirely overcome by love the first time you hold your baby. As much as you love your job, your love for your baby will be completely different. Believe me, there's space in your heart for both.

A big fear of many dads-to-be is that they won't be a good father. Be kind to yourself. You don't have any experience in being a dad. It's so clichéd to say that you should follow your instincts, but it's true. If ever you don't know what to do, remember there can be many people in your life you can ask for advice. This can be a friend who already has kids, your parents, a co-worker, or your baby's doctor. Also, brace yourself now for the unrequested advice even strangers in the park or the mall will be all too happy to hand out. As much as some of these pieces of advice can be helpful, you'll learn to take them with a pinch (or sometimes a whole bag) of salt. What works for some parents might not work for you and your wife. You'll find your own rhythm when it comes to parenting.

A lot of dads-to-be fear they will lose their identity once they become a parent. When your wife reaches the end of her pregnancy and after the baby's born, your free time will become less. This means that you won't have as much time to spend on your favorite hobbies or practicing your favorite sports. A day of golf might now become squeezing in a couple of balls at the driving range if you're lucky. Instead of having your hobbies define who you are, you'll be a dad 24/7. This can change your sense of being; however, this can sometimes even be for the better. Having a baby forces you to mature to the next level, and you'll find other interests involving your child or being a parent. Also, remember that even though being a parent is a lifelong commitment to your child, not having as much time for your hobbies won't be a permanent change. Your child will grow up and become more independent, meaning your time will eventually free up again.

Many parents-to-be (not just dads) will experience a fear of missing out (FOMO), not only while pregnant but possibly for the first couple of years of their child's life. Let's quickly face this truth: You'll miss out on many things. Your life won't be carefree anymore, so you will not be able to drop everything to join your childless friends for a night out or a weekend away. While missing out on those exciting events, you'll gain a new excitement for raising your little human. Seeing your baby take their first step or hearing them say their first word will more than make up for the fun you might have had with friends. Your life will now be filled with memorable, once-in-a-lifetime moments. If you have a sound support system, you also don't have to miss out on seeing the people you care about. Once your child is old enough to sleep out, allow them to spend the night with someone you trust. You'll likely find that you and your wife will enjoy these odd nights out much more than before you had a child, and the following day when you pick the baby up, you'll probably be so happy to see them that you might not even moan about cleaning a dirty diaper.

Lastly, many soon-to-be dads fear getting what is often called the "dad bod." As much as this is a generalized joke, not all fathers pick up extra weight or get a "beer belly." As your family grows, your time for doing exercise will get less. However, if you're strict about being active and not adding any inches around your waistline, you'll be able to achieve this. As your child grows, they will be able to join in your exercise routine. And before that, there's no rule stating you can't use your older baby or toddler as weight. Imagine your child is a 15-pounder dumb-bell, and get those biceps working. Your child's giggles as you lift them up and down might motivate you to do more.

Things All Modern Dads Should Know

Now that you've faced some of the fears keeping you up at night let's delve deeper into your fear of not being a good dad. Just as your wife's body was made to give birth to a baby, your body was designed to be a dad. Want some proof? A study showed specific physiological and neurological changes in a man's body shortly before he becomes a dad (McKay, 2013).

One of the most significant signs is your testosterone levels. To help you become more nurturing, your testosterone levels will drop by about a third around three weeks before your baby's due (McKay, 2013). Don't worry. This won't affect your manliness forever. These levels will rise again to normal levels around six weeks after your baby's birth—coincidently, around the same time, most doctors recommend it is safe for mom to become sexually active again. Happy days are coming! Also, impress your wife with your extensive knowledge by throwing in this fact during a conversation. She'll be impressed, and you'll look like a super dad in the making.

With your testosterone dropping, your brain will become more tuned to a baby's crying as well. This proves the excuse of not hearing the baby crying at night is invalid. Sorry guys!

Also, remember that every dad-to-be handles pregnancy and the birth of their baby differently. While some men are amazed to see their partners pushing the baby through the birth canal, others fear seeing this might have a lasting effect on their desire for their partners. If you fall into this group, don't let that cause you stress. You might be so amazed by what your wife's body is capable of during childbirth that your love and desire for her can shoot through the roof. Remember that you don't have to watch the birth of your baby up close. You can stand by her head and support her through it. When you hear your baby cry, the wonder of childbirth will be over.

If you felt queasy looking at newborn photos online, that is okay. Newborns are often covered with vernix caseosa (the creamy white stuff we'll discuss later), excess hair, and blood. They are not always the picture-perfect sight you'll see in movies. Don't let the fear of being disgusted by the look of your baby freak you out and put you in a negative mindset. The nursing staff will clean all of that off. You might even be so overcome by pride and love for your baby that you won't care how they look. Always remember you're biologically designed to love and care for your baby. The proof is, as we've mentioned in the research.

As you're preparing yourself mentally for the arrival of your baby, parents-to-be need to consider their finances. Speak to friends with babies and ask how their babies have affected their budgets. Look at how much diapers, formula, creams, and other necessities cost and plan how you can fit all of that into your budget. If you need to cut back on certain aspects, start doing this now, so you're used to the changes before your baby's born. If you can, buy some big-ticket items such as a crib, changing table, and pram early on in the pregnancy so you can free up some money closer to when your baby's born. If money is tight, you don't have to buy these items new. Babies use these items for a short time, and you can find preloved items in excellent condition.

While getting yourself ready to be a father, managing your expectations is essential. Not all babies are happy or calm, and some are tiny terrors. Make peace with the fact that your baby might be a little tyrant. If you're mentally preparing yourself for this, your frustration levels will likely be lower when your baby cries for two hours straight than if you expect to have a perfect baby who never cries. I've never heard of a baby who doesn't cry. If your wife births a wonder like this, your baby might just make global news.

Understanding Your Mental Health As a New Dad

Managing your expectations can go a long way in preserving your mental health through this journey of becoming a parent. The fears and worries mentioned above can severely impact a dad-to-be's mental health, so it's important to acknowledge when your mental wellness suffers and to always take care of yourself. Most men will also be reluctant to discuss the decline in their mental health with their partners. How can you moan about your anxiety while your wife's hurling in the toilet from morning sickness (that lasts all day long)? She might even scowl at you mid-vomit, saying something like: You did that to her. Fellas, don't take this personally. She's feeling miserable.

Choose a rare moment where she isn't losing her breakfast, lunch, or supper at the toilet to discuss your fears and anxiety with her. You might be surprised that she'll possibly share many of your worries. She's going through this pregnancy with you and may also feel unsure about how to care for your bundle of joy. Discussing your feelings can, therefore, help both of you.

If you feel that you can't discuss your anxiety with your partner or another friend, it's best to educate yourself as early in the pregnancy as possible, which is why you're reading this. The more you know and understand what is about to happen, the better you'll be able to prepare for it and the less anxiety you'll experience. Think of this as training before a big game. If you train 10 times harder now, you'll be more prepared and confident for the real thing.

Let's look at some of the significant stressors that can increase your anxiety (totally normal, by the way!) over the coming months:

Life changes

All changes can be scary, as it brings a lot of unknown factors. Since becoming a parent is a life-long change, it can provoke even more anxiety. It can be helpful to surround yourself with other dads, as hearing them talk about their experiences can be helpful. You can also look at joining a Facebook group for new dads. They are your knowledge team-mates in this.

Relationship changes

Your relationship with your partner will change. She'll go from not only being your lover but also being a mother. Your child will become her top priority. However, being parents can deepen the bond you two already share. Make sure you talk about things other than her pregnancy and the baby. Make sure you continue to date each other (even if these dates are in your pajamas on the couch at home).

Isolation

Especially during the first months after your baby has been born, you'll rush straight home after work to help your partner with the baby. At least for the first while, you won't be able to meet up with friends at a bar or go to a football game. This isolation can cause anxiety. Before becoming a dad, you were you first, so practice self-care as much as possible. Rope in the grandmas, grandpas, aunts, and uncles to help and escape for some selfish me-time when you need to. Do this for your wife, too, as you'll likely be way less grouchy when you return home.

Being the provider

We've mentioned the financial implications above. Being financially responsible for another life can provoke extreme anxiety. Make sure to plan and budget as much as you can. If need be, save money wherever you can. You might have to make peace with having a beer or two less a week. Have the funeral and mourn the loss of that beer. It'll be okay.

ON A LIGHTER NOTE, now is the time to start memorizing some punchlines. No matter how lame your humor can be, the minute after your baby's born, you'll be officially qualified to tell your "dad jokes." Don't let anyone hold you back; unless your partner gives you a death stare. If so, stop. Immediately.

Creating a Birth Plan

To help ease your anxiety during this time, it can be helpful to start working on your wife's birth plan. This can help reduce the unknown factors increasing your feeling of not having control. You'll soon begin attending prenatal visits to a doctor, so it's important to discuss this birth plan with the healthcare professional. You should also remember that things might not always go exactly according to plan, but that isn't something you should worry about yet.

Discuss the birth plan with your partner to make sure both of your wishes are included there. Once you get closer to the end of the pregnancy, make four copies of the plan: a copy to keep in your wife's hospital bag, another to keep on you, a copy for the doctor, and one for the hospital or center where she'll give birth.

Ask your partner the following questions to compile your birth plan:

- Do you want a home birth? Do you want to deliver at an out-of-hospital birth center? Or do you want to give birth in the hospital?
- Who do you want in the delivery room?
- Do you want to use a specific style of birthing? Examples here can include water, hypnobirthing, or Lamaze.
- If a cesarean section (C-section) is necessary, do you have any specific requests?

- Do you want a birthing coach or doula present?
- Do you want to use pain management? If so, what type of pain management?
- Do you want specific music played during delivery?
- Do you have special lighting requests?
- Who do you want to cut the umbilical cord?
- Do you want the umbilical cord cut as soon as possible, or do you want to delay cutting the cord?
- Are you going to breastfeed the baby? If so, do you want to feed the baby immediately after birth?
- Do you want skin-to-skin contact? Do you want me to do skin-to-skin contact with the baby?
- Do you want to bank cord blood? If so, what arrangements have you made?
- Do you want to keep the placenta? If so, what arrangements have you made?
- Who must be the first person you let know once the baby's born? Add their numbers to the list.
- How do you want to let people know you're parents?

- Will you send a photo to people to announce the birth?
- How long do you want to wait before you allow visitors in?
- Who do you want to visit first?

Once you've completed your birth plan, make copies and prepare them. As the pregnancy progresses, specific aspects of the birth plan might change. Simply make copies again every time things change. It's better to be prepared than to wait for the final draft and only realize on your way to the hospital with a wife in labor that you still need to print it or make copies.

If you have this ready and communicate with the obstetrician-gynecologist (OB-GYN) and hospital, you'll feel much more relaxed and prepared for what is to come. Your anxiety will decrease, and you'll be able to focus on other aspects of the pregnancy, spoiling your wife or sneaking in a quick game with a friend.

Practical New Dad Tip

Talk to your partner as often as possible. It sounds so cliché, but it's never encouraged enough. You're both going through something extraordinary yet utterly uncharted, so communicating your feelings to your partner will help you bond even more. When talking to your partner, be open about what you're feeling and start the conversation with "I" statements, such as "I am feeling nervous about being a bad dad" or "I am scared of not having enough money to care for the baby." This way, you're making yourself vulnerable and opening the conversation so she can either reassure you or let you know she has the same fears and you're not alone.

You can even turn this into a little game where you each take turns saying something you're feeling. This is an excellent way for both of you to discuss things causing anxiety. This will probably start superficially with statements such as, "I am excited about becoming a parent." Make sure to bring some depth in by addressing real concerns. This might make you realize that your partner is also having a rough time. Have lines such as, "I am excited to parent with you," or "I am looking forward to seeing what an amazing mom you'll be," ready to reassure her during these conversations.

If you don't want to start smack-bam with deep feelings or want brownie points, open the conversation with a line like, "I am nervous about what your body will go through during the pregnancy." This way, you're addressing one of your emotions while also showing her that you care about what she's going through. A double win right there!

Be sensitive to her needs during these conversations. Make sure she's comfortable, and don't make a face or sarcastic comment if she interrupts you mid-sentence for yet another pee break. She can't help it. Since she shouldn't be drinking alcohol while pregnant, avoid the urge to crack open a beer for yourself during this talk. Having these types of conversations is something you'll have to learn to do without any liquid courage.

2

SUPPORT HER

Now that we've addressed some of your fears and causes for anxiety, let's turn our focus to the most important person for the next nine months: the mom-to-be. Her body will go through various changes, from raging hormones that result in her turning from your loving wife to a Tyrannosaurus rex within the blink of an eye, the weirdest cravings (think of a hamburger with condensed milk and sardines on it), to having a belly that is about to grow so big that she won't be able to see her toes anymore. How beautiful is it that your child is literally growing inside of her? How freaking cool is that?!

While she's going through all these changes, the fear of childbirth will be ever-present. She'll either have to endure excruciating pain pushing an 8 lb baby out of her vajayjay, or she'll have to undergo major surgery to remove them from her tummy and then be forced to get up and walk around hours after the surgery to care for it. Regardless, I'm sure most women will agree with me; childbirth is no joke.

There will likely be times during the pregnancy when you'll feel powerless, as there isn't much you can do to make any of this easier. However, understanding more about what she's going through mentally, emotionally, and physically will go a long way in ensuring a happy pregnancy for both of you.

Sex and Body Changes During Pregnancy

Let's first discuss the changes that her body will go through. One of the first symptoms she'll probably experience is swollen and painful boobs. Fellas, as attractive as these mamas might look to you, if you value your life, you shouldn't try to touch (or grab) them. Don't even hug her too tightly. Some women feel friskier during the early stages of pregnancy. If you're one of the lucky ones with a partner who always seems ready, enjoy it, but always remember to steer clear of the melons.

Talking of sex, unless there are complications in the pregnancy and your wife's doctor advises against it, it's usually completely safe to be intimate while pregnant. She might not feel up for it throughout the pregnancy and definitely won't want anything close to her fanny after giving birth, so your best chance of getting lucky will be before her tummy starts blowing up. The bigger her belly gets, the less sexy she'll likely feel. Her hormones might also cause her to rarely be in the mood. Sex will also become more uncomfortable as her tummy grows. Never ever make her feel bad if she doesn't feel up to it when you're up.

Another symptom that often manifests early in pregnancy is extreme nausea and vomiting called morning sickness. Don't let the name of this symptom fool you. This doesn't only happen during the morning. Nausea can hit your partner at any time of the day or stick around like a shadow all day, every day. Morning sickness usually shows its ugly head between six to eight weeks of pregnancy. The vomiting can also be completely unexpected, so your wife might throw up in front of you or even in the middle of a busy mall. Never, ever make a face if this happens. She can't help it.

Instead of being disgusted by this (believe me, more disgusting things are waiting for you in the delivery room), help her by stocking up on crackers or ginger biscuits. Both of these are known to decrease the symptoms of nausea. Keep some next to the bed and ensure she eats one the minute she wakes up in the morning before moving around too much. This will help to settle her tummy slightly. If she's feeling sick, never ask her what's for dinner. Man up and cook your own food. Ask her if she wants to eat and, if so, what she wants. Should she be too sick, eat in another room, so she doesn't have to deal with the smell of your food. It might even help you enjoy your meal more, as you won't have to look at her fighting the urge to hurl. If her symptoms get very severe, take her to the doctor. There are many pregnancy-safe medications she can drink to alleviate this symptom. Dehydration is also possible in cases of severe vomiting, which can be dangerous to your wife and the baby. Make sure she drinks enough water!

Apart from what she throws up, you might feel confused by what she wants to eat. These cravings usually start during the first trimester of pregnancy but can peak at any time. They are caused by a combination of hormones, nutritional deficiencies, and an increased sense of taste and smell. Humor her in any weird cravings she might have, and if she sends you out at midnight in search of donuts, be a good guy and get some for her. The couple of minutes of sleep you'll lose going out on the donut run will be worth it. Otherwise, you'll most likely lose sleep due to having a cranky partner in bed with you. Most food cravings are harmless, such as dairy products, fruit, pickles, or chocolate. If the combinations of foods she craves put you off, give her what she wants and leave the room while she enjoys it.

If her cravings are incredibly unhealthy, you can try to beat this by encouraging her to eat a healthy and well-balanced diet. These cravings are often a way for her body to ensure it gets the nutrients, such as iron or calcium, that the baby needs to grow. The cravings might subside if you advocate that she gets in everything she (and the baby) needs. If they are still there, give her what she craves, but keep things in moderation.

When discussing her cravings with her, choose your words carefully. Her hormones are raging, which can result in mood swings severe enough that you might want to run for the hills. Whatever you do, don't run! She's carrying another human being inside her, and her body is trying to figure out what's happening. As much as she tries to, she can't control her hormones or moods most of the time. She might go from being the happiest mom-to-be one minute to crying uncontrollably the next. This is normal, particularly during the beginning and again towards the end of the pregnancy. Share in her excitement when she's happy, comfort her when she's crying (even if it's for no reason whatsoever), and listen while she vents.

If she forgets why she's crying or the cause of her anger is mid-sentence, don't rush to take her to the neurosurgeon for a brain scan or start planning dementia treatment. The hormone surge in her body and physiological changes in her brain can lead to what is often referred to as a pregnancy brain. She might become highly forgetful and struggle to complete tasks. Studies have found that pregnant women have less gray matter volume in the areas of the brain that deal with social skills and building relationships (Barth, 2020). Many believe this is how mama prepares for caring for her tiny human. It's also another pregnancy-related fact you can impress your wife with. You're on a roll here!

Dealing with pregnancy brain can be very frustrating, not just for you but also for your partner. Help her through this by being kind to her and making sure she gets enough sleep, drinks enough water, and plays games that can boost her brain function.

Stress and anxiety can also contribute to her feeling fuzzy and forgetful. Help her to relieve stress by talking with her about her fears, making lists of things that should be done, or giving her massages to help her relax. Who knows what these massages might even lead to... Probably a good night's sleep for you both! I don't know what you were thinking, but not everything has to be dirty or about sex. Come on now, dad-to-be!

Keep Dating Your Wife and Plan a Babymoon

This is the last time you and your wife can go on dates without needing to arrange a babysitter. Soon, you might feel like you're a teenager again, needing to ask your mom (or your babysitter) for permission to go out. Use this time. Plan romantic dates. But do it without having any expectations of a happy ending. Your wife might not be in the mood or too uncomfortable to do the horizontal dance. However, being romantic and showing her that you love and appreciate her will go a long way in improving your odds.

If you want to get the badge of husband of the year, plan a last getaway for just you and your partner before your baby's born. This little vacation is often called a babymoon and will be the last time you can relax together before becoming parents. When planning this getaway, keep your wife's condition in mind. She won't be able to consume any alcohol or sushi or do anything adventurous. Now isn't the time to plan a bungee jumping or deep-sea-diving trip. Your swimmers have done enough already.

Instead, plan activities that both of you can enjoy. This can include a relaxing picnic, a stroll on the beach, sightseeing, or simply spending time indoors in each other's company. All your mom-to-be might want is a king-size bed (for sleeping!), an air conditioner (especially if she's pregnant during summer, as she'll likely feel like a heater), and room service. Alternatively, find out what your wife would like to do.

Make sure you plan this trip well. If you leave it too late during the pregnancy, you'll run the risk of your wife going into labor on location. The last thing either of you will want to do is search frantically for a hospital in a town neither of you knows. She might also develop a pregnancy-related complication causing her doctor to advise her against traveling. No matter when you plan this babymoon during the pregnancy, it'll be good to research that there's a good hospital nearby. Complications during pregnancy can come suddenly and unexpectedly. However, never fear the possibility of complications. You're getting ready with the correct helpful information and tips to be as prepared and confident as possible.

Mental Health During and After Pregnancy

Pregnancy, especially the first couple of months of parenthood, can be a rollercoaster ride, filled with hormones, emotions, and sleep deprivation for you and your partner. As we've mentioned in Chapter 1, this is why it's so important to constantly be looking out for your mental health and seeking the necessary support should you ever find your mental health declining.

The mood swings that come with being pregnant often affect the mental health of the pregnant woman and her partner. She might cry for no reason and get angry over things that usually wouldn't even phase her. This, combined with the stress of becoming a mom, can easily lead to anxiety and depression. The same goes for the dad-to-be. Your sweet wife can now seem like an emotional monster at times. This might cause you to feel helpless and like you can do nothing right.

The slippery slope to mental health issues like depression and anxiety during pregnancy can make this experience even scarier. This is why it's so important to talk as soon as you experience common symptoms, such as extreme stress and worry, sadness, loss of appetite (or sudden overeating), agitation, and lack of interest in things you enjoy.

As much as it's essential to be aware of your mental health during pregnancy, it's even more crucial to take care of yourself after the baby's born. You might have heard "baby blues" or "postpartum depression" before, but it's key to be aware of what exactly this means and what the signs are to look out for so either you or your partner can get the support you might need. Don't feel overwhelmed by the extensive terms and possible scary experiences. Instead, see this as simply becoming aware of the potential effects on your and your partner's mental wellness. Remember that through awareness and education, you gain knowledge and confidence.

Let's first discuss the mental health of the new mom. As much as she's excited about bringing a new life into the world, it might not always affect her as positively as many think. It's also much more common than people realize: One in eight new moms suffer from some sort of postpartum depression (Gomstyn, 2022). As you'll see below, the level of depression a new mom can experience varies from mild to severe.

- Baby blues. This is the most common mental health problem moms deal with after giving birth. The symptoms usually only last for a couple of days to two weeks:
- Sleeping problems
- Irritability
- Lack of concentration
- Anxiety
- Sadness and crying
- Lack of appetite
- Feeling overwhelmed

Postpartum depression. This is often regarded as baby blues when it starts, but the symptoms last longer and can be so severe that they can impair the mom's ability to perform daily tasks or care for the baby. Symptoms of postpartum depression don't always start right after childbirth; they can begin during pregnancy or up to a year of the baby being born:

- Feeling depressed
- Feeling hopeless, inadequate, or worthless
- Isolating from friends and family
- Inability to bond with the baby
- Constant crying
- Lack of energy
- Extreme irritability or anger
- Thoughts of harming herself and/or the baby

Postpartum psychosis. This condition is rare and can have life-threatening consequences if not treated. Symptoms usually start around a week after the baby's born:

- Disorientation and feeling confused
- Paranoia
- Extreme agitation
- Obsessive thoughts, particularly over the baby
- Hallucinations and delusions
- Attempts at harming herself and/or the baby

As mentioned above, postpartum depression can also affect new dads. Similar to how it can affect a new mom, being a depressed new father doesn't mean you're weak or a failure. It's a medical condition called paternal postpartum depression and has the same symptoms as what moms will experience. Research showed that around one in ten new fathers suffers from this mental health condition (Gomstyn, 2022). The following are known to be risk factors for new dads to develop paternal postpartum depression:

- History of depression or other mental health conditions
- Financial difficulties
- Problems in the relationship with your partner
- Being very young

We've already mentioned that having open discussions with your partner can help to alleviate mild symptoms of depression and anxiety. However, if the symptoms last longer than two weeks after the birth of your baby, get worse, or impact your ability to care for your baby, you can benefit from seeking help from your primary care physician. There's no shame in seeking the support you need; instead, the shame lies in believing you don't need help and making this experience even tougher on you than it needs to be. Don't be that guy.

GET help if you need it. Help your partner if she's struggling. Be aware of what is going on and use the knowledge you've gained to act with confidence. The sooner you and your partner get the help you need, the better it'll be for your whole family, especially your new baby.

Practical New Dad Tip

Take your wife out on a date. That might be the last thing on both of your minds, as your thoughts are likely consumed by pregnancy and raising a child. However, that makes this the perfect time to show her you acknowledge how incredible this journey is that you're both embarking on. She'll be carrying your child for nine months. Let her know how absolutely special that is.

3

THE PRE-GAME WARM UP

W ohooo! You now have a much better understanding of what to expect during your wife's pregnancy. You're aware of the changes her body is going through and never question or make remarks about any of her weird cravings. Her boobs are likely only for aesthetic purposes now. If you want to be a star in her life, buy her a bigger bra, as she might need it in the months ahead. You also know that you should always look out for signs of anxiety and depression in her and yourself.

While having overall knowledge of what lies ahead is good, it's just as important to understand the different trimesters of pregnancy and what to expect during each of them. The nine months or forty weeks of pregnancy are divided into three trimesters, although many professionals advocate that the first three months of a baby's life should be regarded as the fourth trimester—another fact you can impress your wife with. Let's start at the beginning and discuss all you should know about the first trimester or the pre-game warm-up of pregnancy.

The First Trimester of Pregnancy

As you might already know or could guess (kudos to you), the first trimester of pregnancy is the earliest stage of pregnancy (or weeks 1 to 13). The weeks of pregnancy are counted from the first date of a woman's last menstrual period before getting pregnant, so the count starts before actually getting pregnant.

Pregnancy symptoms can differ from woman to woman and even from pregnancy to pregnancy. If she's having a tough pregnancy now, it doesn't mean future pregnancies will be the same. In general, the first trimester isn't always the most pleasant time for the mom-to-be. Her body goes through the shock of hormones and drastic changes to get ready to house your tiny human for nine months. As we've mentioned, she might start to experience morning sickness, sore boobs, mood swings, and cravings, but there are many other symptoms associated with the first trimester:

Spotting

Stay calm if your wife comes to you freaking out about bleeding down there. Excessive bleeding can be a sign of miscarriage (we'll discuss that as well), but a degree of slight bleeding can be expected. This is often called implantation bleeding and is simply a result of the embryo implanting in her uterus. Never make a face when she shows you bleeding or other discharge on toilet paper. As gross as it might be for you to see, she's probably freaking out. If there are any concerns about any form of bleeding, it's always best to consult with her doctor.

Discharge

While on the topic of what might show on toilet paper after she wipes, excess discharge is also very common. As long as this discharge is thin and milky, it's perfectly fine. However, call the doctor if it ever turns yellow or green and has a strong smell. Again, avoid calling this discharge "gross" or telling her how badly it smells. Instead, be a good husband and go buy her some pantyliners to help relieve the discomfort any discharge can cause.

Constipation

The hormone increase in her body can slow down the muscle contractions that move food through her digestive system, resulting in excessive gassiness, bloatedness, and constipation. Ensure she eats enough fibers and drinks plenty of water to help with this. Unless your relationship is on that level of comfortableness, never make fun of her or comment on the sound or odor if she farts in front of you. If you value your life and relationship, pretend it never happened.

Fatigue

The first trimester of pregnancy can take a toll on her body, causing extreme fatigue. Let her have a nap while you do some of her household chores. Never make her feel guilty about needing to nap or even comment about the number of naps she has taken in a day. Most importantly, never complain about how tired you might be. Trust me, she's at least 10 times more tired than you.

Frequent urination

Your wife will be peeing a lot more than ever before. Her uterus is expanding rapidly to make space for the growing baby, putting a lot of pressure on her bladder. Make sure your partner doesn't cut down on fluids because of this. Her body will need the fluids to grow your child. Instead, show her you care by stocking up on more toilet paper. If you don't usually use it, go for two-ply. The skin down there will get more sensitive as the pregnancy progresses, so spending a little bit more money on toilet paper will make her life much more pleasant.

Heartburn

This is a common problem many pregnant women complain about during pregnancy, and hormones can again take the blame for this. To help her relieve these symptoms, let her eat smaller meals throughout the day and avoid greasy food. If it gets so bad that she struggles to eat, consult with a doctor. There are many medications she can use that are safe to take during pregnancy.

Baby's Growth

Even though your wife's tummy will likely not show during the first trimester, the changes in her uterus are remarkable. In these few weeks, your baby will go from being a fertilized egg to a fully-formed fetus. The major organs in your baby's body will start to form. Let's look at some of these developments:

The baby's nervous system will begin forming with an open tube from the brain to the spinal cord.

At around six weeks of pregnancy, you might be able to hear the baby's heartbeat on an ultrasound scan. It beats very fast: between 120 to 160 beats per minute (Watson, 2020a). Your heart will likely beat faster with excitement hearing this for the first time.

The baby's soft skeleton begins to grow with a digestive system, including the kidneys and intestines. The lungs will also form but won't fully develop until the third trimester.

The baby can move its muscles, and you'll be able to see this on an ultrasound scan, but your wife won't feel these movements just yet.

Towards the end of the first trimester, your fetus will start to look like a little baby, with a face, tongue, tooth buds, eyelids, fingernails, and genitals. In most cases, these genitals will still be too small to be able to tell the gender of the baby just yet.

By around 13 weeks, your baby will be about 3 in. long (Watson, 2020a).

You should be amazed by reading all of these changes your wife's body creates in the baby. Show this by treating her to something that she really enjoys, even if it's just a quiet, clean, and neat home where she can rest. After cleaning, use this as an excuse to do something you enjoy.

If you want to impress your partner with your extensive knowledge of her pregnancy, there are many places you can get weekly updates on what to expect during that week of her pregnancy and the baby's size and development. You can register on many baby websites to receive weekly emails or download apps on your smartphone to track the pregnancy.

Prenatal Visits, Exercise, and Other Tips

A couple of things should be done during the first trimester. Impress your partner with your knowledge on this, make a to-do list, and take it one thing at a time. The more things you tick off your list, the more you'll be able to relax and enjoy this journey.

At the top of your list should be finding a doctor for your wife. The specialist who deals with pregnancies, childbirth, and postpartum care is an obstetrician, and a gynecologist deals with, amongst others, the reproductive health of women. A doctor who combines both these specialties is called an obstetrician-gynecologist. Get the best of both worlds by listing all the OB-GYNs in your area. By opting for a doctor specializing in both fields, your wife can also build a relationship with this person for future gynecological care.

Unless you live in a small town, you'll likely have a wide variety of OB-GYNs in your area to choose from. Find out which OB-GYNs are in your insurance network if you have health insurance. This will likely narrow your search down. If you have a preferred hospital, look at which specialists have surgical rights there. If your wife's still undecided about who to choose, talk to friends or colleagues who recently had babies about their experiences with their doctors, or search for reviews online.

Remember that the doctor's decision doesn't have to be set in stone. If your wife isn't happy with the chosen doctor, you can always move to another one. Even if you like the chosen doctor, this is about your wife and her care and not about who you prefer. Most OB-GYNs keep availability in their schedules for pregnant women, so you shouldn't struggle too much to get an appointment with a different doctor if need be.

Once your wife decides on a doctor, schedule an appointment. Most OB-GYNs prefer to see their patients toward the end of the first trimester and then every four weeks after that. Try your best to go with her to every appointment. The doctor will do an ultrasound scan at these appointments, so you can see your baby and track its development. The doctor will also check your wife's blood pressure, test her urine for proteins, and weigh her to keep track of weight gain. Fellas, however tempted you might be to sneak a peek at the scale, never ever do this. Soon, your wife will feel enormous and may even feel embarrassed about the weight she's gaining (even though all pregnant women should gain weight). Don't make this experience worse for her by looking. If you accidentally see her weight, never comment about it. If you say something like, "Wow, you're now 30 lb heavier than when we met," you might find yourself single soon. This may seem like common sense, but even common sense isn't always so common. Be her support, not the person who makes her feel uncomfortable or makes fun of her.

Next on the to-do list should be getting an excellent prenatal vitamin for your wife. During the first trimester, it's essential to look for a vitamin containing folic acid (at least 400 micrograms [µg]), as this holds many benefits for the development of your baby's brain and spinal cord (Watson, 2020a). During the second and third trimesters, prioritize that the prenatal vitamin your wife takes is high in omega-3.

If your partner is a smoker, now is a good time to quit this habit. If you also smoke, don't be that guy that smokes around a pregnant woman. As difficult as it might seem, try and quit with her. It won't be easy for her either. Getting rid of this bad habit now will also make this easier once your baby's born, as you don't want to come close to a newborn baby smelling of smoke.

Alcohol is another big no-no while pregnant. If mama craves beer or wine, look for the non-alcoholic options in your local liquor store. She should also cut down on caffeine. It's widely believed that one cup of coffee daily is safe, so make sure one cup is delicious so she can enjoy every sip.

Moderate exercise is important during pregnancy. This will help to keep the mom-to-be healthy, limit excess weight gain, promote your baby's health, and reduce stress and anxiety. Discuss the exercises your wife's planning on doing with her doctor. Especially during the early stages of pregnancy, walking, swimming, yoga, and low-impact aerobics classes are generally considered safe. Things she should avoid are picking up heavy weights and exercises where she might fall. Make this a fun couples activity by joining your wife in working out. It might also be a great bonding opportunity for the two of you; as the saying goes, "A couple who sweat together, stay together." (DiDonato, 2014)

Another thing to consider is breaking the good news to the people you care about. There's no right or wrong time to tell your loved ones. Some people spread the news the minute they get a positive reading on a pregnancy test. Others wait until after their first prenatal doctor's appointment, while many wait to share the excitement at the beginning of the second trimester, as the risk of miscarriage will decrease as the pregnancy progresses. Most companies require pregnant employees to inform human resources by 12 weeks, so remind your wife to double-check the policy at work.

When to Rush to the Doctor

As much as you should never dwell on the negatives, it's essential to be aware of the signs that things might not go as planned. Understanding what to look out for will help you decide when to rush your partner to the doctor or when to put on calming music, give a relaxing massage, or run her a bubble bath.

Heavy bleeding

As we've mentioned above, minor spotting can be perfectly normal. However, if your wife ever experiences heavy bleeding, she should get checked out immediately, as this can signify a miscarriage.

Severe abdominal pain

Some abdominal pain can be expected during pregnancy as ligaments stretch, and her uterus expands to accommodate the growing baby. Should this pain ever become severe or sharp, it's best to have this checked out. This pain can be another sign of miscarriage or an ectopic pregnancy, where the fertilized egg grows outside her uterus.

Dizziness

Severe dizziness can be another sign of an ectopic pregnancy, which can then be a sign of low blood pressure. This is important to notice as if she gets so dizzy, she may faint, and this fall can hurt the baby.

Blurred vision

This can be a sign of gestational diabetes (abnormally high blood sugar) or preeclampsia, a condition caused by high blood pressure that also causes protein in her urine. Both of these conditions can result in severe complications for both your partner and the baby, so it's best to have it checked out.

Deep Dive Emotions

Seeing your baby for the first time on an ultrasound scan and hearing its heartbeat can unlock a whole new flow of emotions: pride, excitement, elation, and the fear that we've discussed. Apart from discussing your emotions and fears, there are many things you and your partner can do together to make sure your mental health doesn't dive during this time:

Eat healthy, regular meals.

Try to do moderate exercise at least three to five times per week.

Be realistic about your expectations of what you, especially your wife, can do. Now isn't the time for her to try and be a superwoman. She's already using all her superpowers to grow the baby and is a real-life wonder woman.

Unless you have to, try not to make significant changes, such as moving house(s), during this time. Keep life as normal and stress-free as possible.

Spend time with the people who are important to both of you, make you happy, and positively impact your life.

If possible, connect with other pregnant couples or couples who recently had a baby. Sharing your experiences and listening to what others went through can be extremely helpful and help to prepare you for all possible events. Keep in mind that not every experience will be the same. Don't let someone else's bad experience make you want to go sit in a dark corner and cry. Your adventure during pregnancy and childbirth might be completely different.

Practical New Dad Tip

Ask your partner what food she's craving or what she absolutely doesn't want anywhere close to her. Her body and hormones are changing, so letting her know you acknowledge that by asking what she wants to eat is an excellent way to support her and make her feel loved and appreciated.

4

THE FIRST HALF

Boom! You've made it to the honeymoon stage of the pregnancy. The second trimester is usually considered the most fun for both mom and dad. The extreme sickness and fatigue she might have felt during the first trimester will soon be gone, and she'll have a couple of weeks' break before the extreme uncomfortableness of the growing baby will get her down during the third trimester. Now is a great time to go on that babymoon we discussed in Chapter 2.

Over the next couple of weeks, you will, if you choose to know, likely find out the gender of the baby. The baby's movements will also get stronger. First, your wife, and then you can feel the baby's kicks. Your wife's tummy will also grow, and the preggy belly will become more and more noticeable. Now is the time to work on bringing your A-game regarding guard duties. Strangers might randomly start touching your wife's tummy. This strange phenomenon will only get more extreme once the baby's born, as some will try to touch your precious tiny human. Keep your pimp hand strong and ward off any unwanted affections.

You Made It Through the First Trimester

Your partner has made it through the pre-game warm-up and is now in the first half, AKA the second trimester of the pregnancy. This trimester starts in week 14 and continues until week 27. Although some bad symptoms, such as heartburn, your wife will likely start to feel much better and more energetic. Her boobs will probably also not be so sore anymore, and her increased estrogen levels might work in your favor, so your luck in getting her frisky might be up.

Since her energy levels should be up and her belly growing, why not take her on a nice shopping trip for maternity clothes? Her clothes won't fit for much longer, and if you wait till her tummy is peeking out her shirts, she might be too sore and uncomfortable to walk around in the mall. Help her on this trip. Don't stand around irritated at the shops' entrances or mall aisles waiting for your wife to get done. Help her to choose clothes, or surprise her with something she likes later at home.

As your baby grows, its movements will become more significant. Between 18 to 25 weeks, your wife will start to feel these movements. At first, it'll feel like fluttering but will soon become proper kicks. Only a couple of weeks after your wife starts to feel the first movements, you'll also be able to feel the karate kid's kicks. When looking at the week-by-week milestones during pregnancy, always keep in mind that every pregnancy progresses at its own pace. Yours might not be exactly as it is believed to be, so if you're ever concerned about milestones not being reached, discuss this with your OB-GYN.

Towards the end of the second trimester, your partner may start to struggle to get comfortable enough to fall asleep. Here are two more chances to impress your wife. Firstly, advise her to sleep as much as possible on her left side, as this increases the blood flow to her uterus. Secondly, and this can be quite an award-winning move for you, buy her a pregnancy pillow. This long, C-shaped pillow supports her head, neck, and growing belly and back. After the baby is born, this pillow can be just as handy for them to lay on during feeds. However, as the baby gets bigger, pack this pillow far away. Otherwise, your wife might just start to love and cuddle it more than you.

As the pregnancy progresses, you might notice changes in your partner's skin. Due to the increase in hormones, she might feel like she's a teenager again struggling with acne. Stretch marks may appear soon, particularly on her tummy, breasts, and bum. Never comment on these stretch marks; see them as another reminder of the miracle her body is busy creating. Vitamin E oil can help to reduce the appearance of these marks and is safe to use during pregnancy.

She might also develop dark marks on her face called melasma and a dark line down the middle of her stomach called linea nigra. These changes should fade and eventually disappear after the baby's born. Apart from this, her skin will become more sensitive. Make sure to rub her with sunscreen that has an SPF of at least 30 when she goes outside.

Towards the end of this trimester, your partner can experience pains in her lower abdomen. This is due to her expanding uterus, which puts extra pressure on and stretches her ligaments and muscles. She might also have backache(s) caused by the excess weight she's carrying around her belly. Take out the vitamin E oil and use it again to give her a relaxing massage.

Many pregnant women experience bleeding gums, and this is due to hormones causing the gums to swell. If your wife suffers from this, get her a tooth-brush with softer bristles to use in the meantime, and remind her to be gentler when she flosses her teeth. Nosebleeds are also more common during pregnancy, as the hormones can cause the mucus membranes in the nose to swell. This can even cause your wife to start snoring. Don't mock her for snoring. Help her by getting a pregnancy-safe decongestant or saline drop to alleviate the buildup in her nose.

The second trimester is a good time to look into birthing or antenatal classes. This will help you prepare for what to expect in the delivery room, how to help your wife through labor, what will happen after your baby's birth, and how to care for your baby once you take your new family member home. Most importantly, this will help you realize you won't break the baby by picking them up, that it's perfectly fine and manly to be goofy around your child, and that you're allowed to brag as much as possible.

If you want to up your fatherly game now, look into how to take the best photos or videos of a newborn. Mom will be busy nursing or caring for the baby, and one of your first jobs will be to take as many photos as possible. Eventually, photos, videos, and your memories will be all you'll have of your baby's first couple of days, so make sure not to fumble your first duties of fatherhood. Instead, secure yourself a badge of honor by capturing the first days as best you can.

Size of Your Baby

While your wife's experiencing all these changes, your baby's growing at a steady pace. Many of the baby's organs are now fully formed, and the baby can swallow, suck, open their eyelids, hiccup, and hear your voice. By this stage, your baby will even have its own fingerprints. The baby will start to go through cycles of being awake and sleeping.

Since your baby's in amniotic fluid, fine hair called lanugo, and a vernix caseosa, a creamy, white coating covers the baby's entire body. This protects the baby's skin from being constantly in the fluid. This vernix is absorbed by the skin, and babies born after their due date will likely not have any traces of vernix on their skin at birth.

By the end of the second trimester, your baby should be around 3 pounds and 16 inches long, around the size of an English cucumber (Watson, 2020b).

Baby's Gender

Finding out the gender of your little bundle of joy is another exciting part of pregnancy. Some people prefer to wait until the baby is born and get the surprise in the delivery room, while others want to find out what they are expecting as soon as possible. Knowing what you're expecting can make it easier to prepare for the baby's arrival if you want to use traditional gender colors in the baby's room or clothes.

Unless the baby's in a difficult position during your ultrasound scan, most OB-GYNs can determine the gender of the baby between 16 to 20 weeks, although it can sometimes be seen on the scan as early as 14 weeks. The OB-GYN will generally look for the presence of a penis. If a penis can be seen on the scan, the doctor will quickly tell you it's a boy. However, this isn't always accurate. If your baby's a late bloomer, or if the penis is hidden behind the umbilical cord or between the legs, you might think you're expecting a girl, only to get the surprise later on.

Tell the doctor if you want to keep the baby's gender a surprise. Should you wish to find out, decide how you'd like this to happen. Some couples ask the OB-GYN to tell them during an ultrasound scan, while others want to find out surrounded by the people they care about during a gender reveal party.

If you want to do a party, you can ask your OB-GYN to write the gender of the baby on a piece of paper, closed in an envelope. This can then be handed to whoever is helping to keep the gender secret. Some people like to put either blue or pink feathers in a dark balloon that the pregnant couple must pop to reveal the gender, while others have a color-themed cake made, where the gender is revealed once the cake is cut. However you decide to do it, make sure you have the right equipment. You don't want to stand forever trying to pop a balloon with a blunt needle. It's also best not to have this balloon filled with helium, as you might accidentally release the balloon into the sky while still getting ready to pop it. If this happens while a family member records you, you might become the butt of a joke going viral on social media.

Apart from seeing the penis (or lack of a penis) on the ultrasound scan, other tests can help to identify the gender. Since these tests are often not done routinely and can carry some risks, most OB-GYNs wouldn't advise doing them simply to determine the gender of the baby. These tests include:

Amniocentesis

This is done to detect developmental issues in a fetus, such as Down syndrome and spina bifida. A long needle is inserted into the womb to withdraw amniotic fluid. Tests done on this fluid can show the gender of the baby. It does, however, bring a risk of miscarriage, so it's only done if there's a significant concern over the baby's development.

Chorionic villus sampling

This is another test done to diagnose Down syndrome in an unborn baby. Through this test, a sample of the placenta is removed. It shows the genetic information of the baby, which includes the gender of the baby. This test also carries the risk of miscarriage and preterm labor.

Non-invasive prenatal test

This blood test checks for the possibility of a chromosomal disorder. It's usually done if you're at high risk of giving birth to a baby with a chromosome abnormality.

Practical New Dad Tip

Ask your partner if she'd like to do a gender reveal party. It can be a great way to bring the families together and celebrate another milestone for your soon-to-be little human. Decide whether you want to arrange this party yourself or if you want to ask a family member or friend to host it. Remember to make sure the way you'll reveal the gender is foolproof.

5

THE SECOND HALF

The home stretch of the pregnancy! The first trimester, stretching from weeks 28 to 40, or whenever the baby's born, can be the most taxing on the mom-to-be. To say she'll be uncomfortable will be the understatement of the century. Even though this last trimester is only 12 weeks, it'll feel like a year for her.

Her tummy will be huge, her legs will likely swell, she'll be tired from running to the bathroom all the time, and as much as people will advise her to sleep before the baby comes, she'll struggle for most of the night to get comfortable enough to fall asleep. If she does get comfortable, she'll likely only get to lay like that for a minute or two before she needs to rush to the bathroom for yet another pee break. Your baby will be using her bladder as a trampoline, bouncing around in her uterus like a true gymnast. Every time this happens, your wife will need to run (or waddle) to the bathroom as soon as possible.

If things ever get so rough that you feel like drowning yourself in the toilet bowl, remind yourself that in only a couple of weeks, everything you've been going through will be worth it. Soon you'll be parents and hold your tiny human in your arms.

What to Expect in Your Third Trimester

Women in their third trimester of pregnancy are generally highly uncomfortable. The baby's growing fast and will start to move closer to the birth canal, making it even more difficult for her to get comfortable. Imagine trying to force a watermelon through a hosepipe. This is what, in essence, will be going on inside her body. She'll struggle to do her chores around the home. Help her in any way she can. Do the laundry, clean the house, do the dishes, and make supper. The less she has to do, the more she'll be able to (at least try to) rest. She'll need all her energy for labor and childbirth.

Speaking of energy, if she gets up with the urge to clean one day, know that the end of the pregnancy is getting very close. This is called nesting and means her motherly instincts are letting her know it's time to make sure everything is ready for the baby's arrival. Many women experience this a day or two before they go into labor. If this nesting urge hits your partner, don't try and stop her. Her efforts will only cause an argument and won't get her to stop. Instead, help her as much as possible without getting in her way.

If you haven't yet gotten the baby's room ready, don't wait any longer. You'll bring your tiny human home in only a couple of weeks. Make sure everything's ready. Look at getting a changing table at a comfortable height so you and your partner won't have to bend over every time you change your baby's diaper. Look at getting a crib and a comfortable chair for feeding the baby. This will be particularly handy during nighttime feeds. You should also look for a car seat and a pram to bring the baby home safely. Decide on what you really need before you set foot in a baby store. There's a lot of equipment on the market that babies rarely use, and unless you have the financial means to splurge on items that will be used only once or twice, make sure of what you truly need. The sales staff at your local baby store will try to convince you to buy much more than you actually can afford and will use. Be strong, and don't fall for their sweet smiles and "friendly" advice. It's all just sales tactics.

Apart from being uncomfortable, she'll experience more pain leading to the end of the pregnancy. The ligaments and muscles in her tummy will be stretched to the extreme. She'll have backache(s) most days due to the extra weight she's carrying around. Her feet might get swollen, causing pain when she has to walk. The lower the baby drops into the birth canal, the more pain she'll experience in her pelvic area. Some women even describe having sharp stab-like pains in their vajayjays. This is all normal. Giving her a massage can help to alleviate some of these aches, or get her heating pads. You'll seem super caring for doing this—brownie points! Otherwise, let her relax on a comfortable couch and serve her when you're at home. Even if she doesn't say or show it, she'll appreciate any help she can get.

As the pregnancy progresses, she might start to experience Braxton Hicks contractions. These are mild and irregular contractions, helping her body practice for the real deal. They are mostly just uncomfortable and can cause a slight tightness in her abdomen. The closer she gets to her due date, the more intense these practice contractions can become. Braxton Hicks causes many women to rush to the hospital, thinking they are in labor. If you know and understand the difference between Braxton Hicks and true labor, you won't only be able to calm your wife down and avoid rushing her to the hospital but also impress her with your extensive knowledge. Another partner-of-the-year award is loading!

The easiest way to determine if her contractions are Braxton Hicks or true labor is to let her walk or move. Braxton Hicks tends to go away as soon as the mom-to-be moves, whereas true labor will only stop once the baby has been born. Another way to determine what you're dealing with is to time it. True labor contractions will be regular and intensify in strength and frequency, while Braxton Hicks will be irregular and become weaker until they fade completely. Braxton Hicks will only be felt in her abdominal area, whereas true labor can be felt in the abdomen and lower back.

As the baby moves down into your wife's pelvis and becomes engaged in the birth canal, she'll become even more of a urine machine than ever before. The baby, placenta, and uterus will be pushing on her bladder, causing her to pee much more than ever before. The pressure of the dropping baby can cause your wife to swell down there, stretching her skin. Remember the two-ply toilet paper that I advised you to buy? If you haven't done that yet, now is the time. The stretched skin can quickly become sore and irritated, particularly with all the wiping from frequent toilet trips.

If you want to take your partner on one last date before the baby's arrival, be sure to take her somewhere, she'll be comfortable and won't have to walk a lot. Taking her for a meal and/or watching a movie can be a good way for her to relax. If you opt for a movie, book your tickets early enough to ensure you can get an aisle seat for her, as she'll probably have to make a couple of loo breaks during the movie. If you have a cinema close to you with recliner chairs, spend a little bit of extra money on that cinema, as these will be much more comfortable for her. When choosing a movie, keep in mind that this date is to spoil her, so choose something she'll enjoy and want to see. Research the film's running time beforehand, as you don't want to take her to watch something three hours long. Even in the most comfortable recliner chair, she'll get uncomfortable sitting for that long.

You can also look at treating her with a pedicure, either by yourself or at a salon or spa. With her growing tummy, there will be no way she'll be able to safely reach her sore feet and toes for the care she deserves. During labor, her feet will likely be on display in stirrups. Her dogs will be out! Make sure she doesn't feel ashamed of the condition of her feet. While we're on the topic of personal care, help her out by shaving her legs, and if this is what she prefers, trim or shave her vajayjay as well. It has likely been a couple of weeks since she was last able to see down there, and even with all the mirrors in the world, she'll struggle to clean up the downstairs area. Her vagina will be the main attraction during labor, so help her so that it's in the condition she prefers.

It's good to practice your go-to answer for questions such as "Do I look fat?" or "Is my tummy huge?" If you have answers ready for these trick questions, you can answer quickly with a smile and without hesitation. A suggested answer will be something like, "Absolutely not. You're beautiful."

Lastly, as she reaches full-term pregnancy, she might become desperate to start labor. Old wives' tales want people to believe that drinking castor oil or eating Vaseline can help to bring on labor. However, medical professionals advise against this, as it can cause serious harm to the mom-to-be and the unborn baby. She can try many safer options, such as walking, bouncing carefully on a yoga ball, or eating spicy food (best to avoid this if she's struggling with heartburn). Another option that has some scientific backing, is sex. The theories as to why this might be the preferred go-to to get labor kickstarted include:

- Having an orgasm can help to stimulate the womb into starting true labor contractions.
- Your semen can help to ripen the opening of her cervix.
- Sex, particularly nipple stimulation, triggers the release of oxytocin, the same hormone that helps bring on contractions.

If you explain these possible benefits to your partner, it might increase your odds of getting lucky. And, of course, you'll sound highly knowledgeable. Should your partner agree to try this, take your time in finding a position that will work for her, and work around the big tummy as much as possible. If she doesn't feel up to this, never put any pressure on her. She's extremely uncomfortable and a fantastic mama already growing your tiny human. Be kind to her at all times. She's exhausted.

There are, however, instances where sex will become an absolute hard no. This will be after her water breaks, if she has placenta praevia (low-lying placenta—your OB-GYN will inform you during an ultrasound scan if this is a problem), or if she has any bleeding. It's always best to discuss this with your OB-GYN to avoid your penis causing any harm to your new family member.

Your Baby's Development

By the time your wife reaches the third trimester of pregnancy, the baby's significant development has been completed. Their lungs are more mature but won't be able to breathe until around 36 to 38 weeks.

They will, however, start to practice breathing around week 32. Since all the other major organs will be ready for your baby to survive outside the womb, your baby will now start to gain weight (and do this quickly) to make sure they have enough fat in their little bodies to keep them warm after birth.

The baby's pupils will become reactive to light, and their bones will harden. They will be able to suck their thumbs and cry. The lanugo, or layer of downy hair on their bodies, will start to disappear, and their skin will absorb the vernix caseosa, that white, creamy layer protecting their skin from the amniotic fluid. By the time they reach their due date, the average baby is 20 in. (50 cm) long and weighs about 7.5 lb (3.4 kg) (Healthdirect Australia, 2020).

Even though pregnancy is generally 40 weeks long, the baby's considered full-term from week 37 onwards. Some pregnancies last longer than 40 weeks. Generally, your OB-GYN will look at inducing labor if it has not started naturally by 42 weeks.

Your Child's Almost Here! Think About a Name

Naming your child will be one of the greatest decisions you'll make. It's a decision that your child will carry with them for their entire life, so carefully consider this. You might feel pressure from family members to continue the family legacy names, but ultimately, what you decide to name your child has got nothing to do with anyone but you and your partner. Let's look at some of the things you might want to consider when deciding on a name:

Forget the trends

Many people use the latest trends to decide on a name for their child. Too often, these trends pass quickly, and your child might be stuck with a name that might sound ridiculous in a couple of years. When wanting to use a trend as a name, think about how this name will sound in 10 or 20 years time. Will your child have to explain how their parents got this name daily? Will this name embarrass your child? Maybe you'll realize that naming your child born in the middle of the NFL season "Footie" might not be the best idea.

Think about the spelling

Misspelling names on purpose is another thing to carefully consider. Instead of going for the traditional "Rebecca," some opt to spell their children's names "Rabhekkha" or "Rybecka." Although there's nothing wrong with changing the spelling of your child's name, consider how often they would have to spell their names to others and how often their child's name might get mispronounced.

Consider the classics

Some names have been around for centuries, and there's a reason for that. As boring as the classics might seem, deciding on a name that has stood the test of time will ensure your child won't have to explain this name, spell it out, or have it mispronounced.

The family tree

If you decide you want to use a family name for your child, there's nothing wrong with it. However, you don't necessarily have to go for the most immediate family name. Look back at the names of your great-grandparents. There might be something golden hiding way up high in your family tree.

Look at your culture or religion

Opting to honor your culture or religion in your child's name can be a good idea. If you follow the Christian religion, there are many gems of names in the Bible, such as Noah, Luke, Hannah, and Eve. Exploring your culture and religion might just help you find the winner.

Research the meanings

Before you settle on a name, make sure it has the meaning you think it has. Many people might not know that the name "Cameron" means crooked nose. This name is of Scottish origin, and according to the native Scottish Gaelic language, *cam* is translated to "crooked," and *sròn* means "nose." It's believed that the name originated as a nickname given to a member of a Highland clan who obviously had a real looker of a nose. As much as the funny or weird meanings of names aren't always known, these hidden meanings tend to come out on the school playground. So, either make sure there are no funny hidden meanings or practice a one-liner with your child to shut up any possible mockers.

Think about nicknames

While we're on the subject of school ground mocking, consider all possible nicknames your child might have based on their names. An excellent example is Richard, who is often called "Dick." Carefully consider if this is what you want for your innocent bundle of joy. Again, if you're set on this name, help your child with appropriate comebacks to any mocking.

Look at the initials

If you decide to give your child more than one name, write out the initials of the chosen names to make sure it doesn't spell anything funky. Your child might end up being "Lily Olivia Leah" (L. O. L.), "Frederick Michael Lucas" (F. M. L.), or "Ashley Steven Shaun" (A. S. S.). Not being careful of this might scar your child for life.

To use a middle name or not

Even though you should be careful with the initials of your child's name, using a middle name can be an easy way to deal with the pressures of using a family name. Instead of naming your child, for example, Nicholas XI, use Nicholas as a second name and go wild with picking your favorite name to actually call your child.

Say it

Once you've narrowed down your choices, say the names with your last name to hear how it sounds. Your initial favorite might soon be less of a favorite. An example of this is calling your daughter Addison Jackson. It might seem like a good idea, but hearing it, you might feel like there are just too many *sons* in it. If you have family members with strange accents, also consider how your child's name will sound when they say it. This can also put a damper on your original favorite.

Do more research

It can help to do a thorough online search of your favorite names to see where they may have been associated with a villain or someone with a bad reputation. Suddenly, the name Joseph might remind you of Joseph Stalin, or naming your baby Ursula will remind you of The Little Mermaid every time you call her. There might even be a porn star using the exact same name and surname. This might also be something you want to consider avoiding.

Choose a Godparent or Guardian

Another big decision you and your wife will have to make is deciding who to ask to be your baby's godparents or guardians. **Godparents** traditionally fill a spiritual role in your baby's life. If you're religious, they will be responsible for making sure your child is brought up understanding your religion and the higher power or God you pray to. Unless you specifically name them as your child's legal guardian in your will, they will only be there to guide your child, not to take care of your child should you and your partner be unable to.

. . .

GUARDIANS WILL BE the ones taking over the role of your child's parents in the event of death or incapability. As mentioned above, a guardian must be named in your will. It's always best to discuss your wishes with your chosen guardians in case of an unfortunate event. This is probably one of the most important decisions you'll make as a parent.

So, in short, your child doesn't necessarily need to have a godparent if you aren't religious or don't see the need for one, but all children should have a legal guardian specified in their parents' will. Otherwise, your child could be left in the state's care, who will then decide on an appropriate person to care for your child.

Whether you're choosing a godparent or guardian for your child, the same critical factors should be considered:

Make sure the person will be there for your child

In general, most parents choose to appoint someone who is family, as they are likely to be involved in your child's life for the long haul. Should you go for a friend, make sure you have a long, solid relationship, and should quarrels ever arise, sort any issue out as soon as possible. There's no point in having someone as your child's godparent or guardian if your child doesn't know them and they haven't been part of their life. The new buddy you might have made at the bar shortly before your wife became pregnant is probably not the ideal person to ask to play this role in your child's life.

Consider the influence they will have on your child's life

Think about the moral values of these people. Are they kind? Do they show respect to others? What will they teach your child? Do they have a similar type of lifestyle to yours? These factors are often just as important as whether they will have the financial means to care for your little one. It might sound like common sense, but these are all essential things to consider and think over with your partner.

Make sure you choose your child's godparents or guardians for the right reasons

Often a best friend or sibling will expect you to select them. However, pleasing these people might not be in your child's best interests. Instead, choose someone you trust with your life, as you will, in essence, hand over your life to them should something happen to you.

Have a frank discussion with your chosen godparents or guardians about expectations

Tell them exactly what you want them to do and what type of role you want them to play in your child's life. Similarly, they should explain their expectations as well. In the case of guardians, they might want to know what type of financial provisions you're making for your child. Play open cards with them, and should you decide to take out policies for your child, make sure the guardians have all the details of these policies and any pension funds or other savings you might have.

NEVER TAKE it to heart if your chosen godparent or guardian declines the invitation. They might have personal reasons why they don't feel they should accept this responsibility. If you want, ask them to still play an important but unofficial role in your child's life. Should you decide to name either your parents or your in-laws to be the guardians, make sure to revisit this decision annually. They will get older and might become incapable of looking after a young child. So as much as they might be the ideal choice now, they might not be as suitable in a couple of years' time.

Practical New Dad Tip

If you want to buy new furniture for your home, carefully consider what you'll buy. Your baby might do a number on the new couch you buy, so it doesn't have to be the prettiest or whitest piece of furniture.

Wake up early on a Saturday morning before your wife pops your soon-to-be baby and go garage sale hunting. You'd be surprised how many people would practically give away their furniture to you for great bargains. Also, Craigslist has a free section where people give away all kinds of items every week. It's worth checking both of these out. And I bet your pregnant partner will be happy that you scored such a great deal.

6

YOU'RE IN DOUBLE OVERTIME

W ifey has reached the end of the pregnancy. The moment you've both been waiting and preparing for over the past nine months is getting closer by the day. Now it's time to have your game face on and be ready for whatever can happen during this double-overtime phase.

To make sure you're ready, we'll go over every step, including what to take with you to the hospital, when to go to the hospital, what to expect in the delivery room, what will happen during a C-section if your wife will need one, and any other possibilities that can occur during the birth of your child. It's go time!

What to Pack for the Hospital

Once your partner starts experiencing Braxton Hicks contractions, it's good to pack the bags to take with you to the hospital, so you're ready for when the real deal comes. This will include everything your partner and baby will need during and after the birth, as well as snacks for yourself during the delivery. When getting everything together for your partner and the baby, prepare for at least a four-day stay. If the baby's born via natural vaginal birth, you'll likely bring your new family home the next day. However, if there are complications or your baby's born via a cesarean section, their hospital stay can extend to a couple of days. The average length of a hospital stay post-C-section is two to four days. Be prepared for this.

Helping a mom-to-be in labor and caring for a brand-new life will likely make you run around like a chicken with its head cut off. Don't add any more stress by not packing everything you'll need. It can be good to leave a copy of your house keys with a trusted family member or friend. This way, you can ask them to bring anything you might have forgotten to the hospital instead of driving up and down when your partner needs you the most.

To help you up your game in your new daddy role, I've included checklists of everything that should be packed for the hospital.

Mom's Bag for Delivery

This bag will contain everything your wife might need during labor. Remember that labor can easily last for numerous hours, especially with a first pregnancy.

Paperwork

Many hospitals require the mom-to-be to register and book a bed at the hospital. If that is the case, most of the paperwork will be sorted out before the delivery. Whether this is the case or not, make sure you have any necessary medical records, your wife's ID, and your health insurance card ready when you take your laboring wife to the hospital. You'll likely be expected to open her file at admissions after you take your wife to the delivery room. Make this trip to admissions as short as possible by having all possible documents ready.

Her birth plan

We've discussed the birth plan already. You might have handed in a copy of the birth plan by the hospital beforehand. Whether this was the case or not, make sure to bring a copy with you to the hospital. If your partner's labor progresses fast, there will be no time for the hospital staff to search for her birth plan. Have it ready.

Bathrobe

The hospital will give your wife a theater gown to put on while in labor. These gowns are not exactly glamorous or comfortable. Most are open at the back. During labor, the nurses might advise your wife to walk around the ward to help her labor progress. Don't let her walk around with her bum exposed. She'll already feel like she's a part of an interactive museum exhibition by the way the nursing staff will look at her vajayjay and check how far her cervix has dilated using their gloved hands.

Let her keep the little bit of dignity she might still have left by keeping her behind covered.

Socks

During labor, the blood flow in her body will change, with her body directing the focus toward her contracting uterus. This can result in her feet feeling cold. Pack thick socks in the bag, so she's warm and comfortable.

Slippers

Since the mom-to-be might be advised to walk around the labor ward, remember to pack slippers to reduce the risk of her slipping and hurting herself or the baby. Make sure she can put these slippers on easily by herself and that they don't fit too tightly on her swollen feet.

Lip balm

During labor and delivery, her lips might get chapped. Giving her some lip balm will bring her much-needed relief.

Face cloth

Many women feel extremely hot during delivery and will sweat profusely. Pack a face cloth to help her through this. Be the best husband by keeping this face cloth (moist and cool, of course) in hand during delivery to place on her face or forehead to cool her off.

Hair ties and clips

If your wife sweats during delivery, she might get irritated by hair hanging on her face, making her feel even hotter. In what can only be described as a superman moment, you can take out hair ties and clips and show your quick instincts by gently tying her hair back. Then, give yourself a quick pat on the back for remembering to bring these before surrendering your hand back to her (not-so-merciful) squeezes.

Entertainment

As we've said, labor can take hours. Pack some entertainment for both of you. This can be magazines or books or downloading her favorite shows or podcasts onto a device to watch. This can help distract her from what her body is going through while keeping her mind off how long labor is taking.

Her preggy pillow

The hospital will give her pillows, but these might not be the most comfortable. Try and help her by taking her preggy pillow (or favorite pillow) with you to the hospital. She might not be able to take it to the delivery room but can use it in the labor ward and after the baby's birth.

Mom's Bag for After Birth

After your wife has shown her true Wonder Woman spirit by giving birth to your baby, make sure she feels at home during the rest of her hospital stay. Remember to pack enough clothes and toiletries for at least a four-day stay.

Comfortable pajamas

Whether she gives birth naturally or via cesarean section, she'll want to feel as comfortable as possible afterward. Pack her favorite pajamas or treat her to new ones. If she plans to breastfeed, make sure the pajama top can open in the front. Opt for pajamas darker in color, so she isn't overcome with embarrassment should she fill her maternity pad so quickly that blood leaks onto her pajamas. Since babies can't generate their own body heat, the temperatures in maternity wards are typically kept quite warm. She'll also handle the baby, covered in warm blankets, often. Make sure to pack cooler pajamas for her additionally, so she doesn't get too hot.

Nursing bras.

If she breastfeeds the baby, nursing bras will be a lifesaver for her. On these bras, the cups open in the front, creating easy access to release the nipple for feeds. If she opts to feed the baby formula, ensure she has comfortable bras, as she wouldn't want the girls hanging loosely when visitors come. Now isn't the time to wear lace push-up bras. Cotton bras without any underwires will likely be most comfortable.

Extra underwear

After giving birth, she'll bleed more than a year's worth of periods combined. This might cause her to leak onto her underwear. Make sure she has enough spare underwear to change regularly.

Maternity pads

Speaking of blood, she'll need maternity pads for the first couple of days after birth. These pads look more like surfboards than regular protective products. Never mention the size of them. Just hand her one without making any type of face when she needs one. In case of severe bleeding or during the night, it can help to double-pad. Give her this tip to show you're not grossed out by it.

Breast pads and nipple cream

If she opts for breastfeeding, pack her some breast pads. This will absorb any milk leakage, so she doesn't sit with embarrassing wet marks on her pajama tops. Breastfeeding, especially at the beginning, can be extremely painful. She and her baby will learn to find the best ways for the baby to latch.

This process can result in severely sore and even cracked nipples. Using a nipple cream can reduce the pain she'll experience.

Toiletries

Any toiletries she'll use on an ordinary vacation trip, she'll need in the hospital. This includes soap or shower gel, shampoo, conditioner, face wash, toothpaste, toothbrush, hairbrush, hair ties or clips, deodorant, and whatever else she might use.

Charger

Many couples forget to take phone chargers with them. Your phone's battery will deplete quickly due to all the photos taken, phone calls, and messages received. Remember to also take an extension cord in case the plug in her ward is far from her bed. An extension cord can help her use her phone while sitting comfortably on the bed.

Clothes

Even though she'll likely be in pajamas during her hospital stay, she'll need a clean set of clothes for when she's discharged, and you take her home. If she has had a C-section, make sure these clothes are comfortable and loose-fitting, as the cut on her abdomen will be sore.

Snacks and drinks

The hospital will provide her with meals, but she might want some comfort food after giving birth. Pack as many of her favorite snacks as you can fit in the bag. Remember to also pack some water or juice, especially if she's going to breastfeed, as feeding her baby can dehydrate her quickly.

Your Bag for Delivery

As we've mentioned, labor can take a good number of hours. Make sure you take everything you'll need to make it as comfortable and pleasant as possible for you.

Snacks and drinks

You'll get hungry during labor, and you don't want to have to run to a shop every time you feel like having a snack or a drink of water. Pack enough snacks for you and your wife. If your wife's doctor advises that she shouldn't eat, don't be that guy to eat in front of her, even if she says it's okay. Believe me, it's not okay. Have a bite of something while you're in the passageways on a phone call or while the doctor is busy examining your wife.

Clothes

You won't know how long you'll be in the hospital for labor, so it's always the safest option to take an extra set of clothes. You also don't know what might happen during delivery. I don't want to freak you out, but many women experience nausea and vomiting due to the extreme pain from labor. Your wife might vomit while you're still helping her to the bathroom, leaving you in the firing line. Surprisingly, being vomited on will probably not be the last time you're around an exchange of fluids that day. And, with a newborn at home, it'll definitely not be the last time someone will vomit on you. Embrace this new part of fatherhood, and change clothes as soon as your wife's safely back in bed.

Pillow

Since labor can take a good couple of hours and the chairs in the labor ward might not be the most comfortable, taking a pillow with you might be helpful. Rest while you can, especially during the beginning of labor. Once the labor intensifies, there will be no rest for either of you. Imagine an all-nighter on steroids!

Toiletries

After the baby's born and your wife's safely in the maternity ward with your newborn, you might want to freshen up quickly. Take some toiletries for yourself, even if it's just a toothbrush.

Phones, cameras, batteries, and chargers

Remember what we said about your first duty as a new father being that of a photographer or videographer? Don't forget to pack the equipment you might need. If your phone takes good photos, make sure your phone is fully charged before your partner is moved from the labor ward to the delivery room. If you're going to use a camera, pack extra batteries.

You don't want to miss a single moment of what is to come.

Entertainment

Here is a *big* and *important* note: Only watch some Netflix while your wife doesn't need your help and is in the labor ward. The minute your wife moves to the delivery room, you shouldn't even touch your phone unless she wants you to record the delivery. Otherwise, pick up your phone or camera after your baby has been born to take photos.

Baby's Bag

After you've packed all the other bags, it's now time to think about what your baby will need. Now is also a good time to make sure the baby's car seat is installed in your car. Practice exactly how to use it. This might sound ridiculous; how hard can it be to click the clips in right? Well, you'd be surprised just how much you might struggle with this seemingly simple task when you have to secure a crying baby in it for the first time.

Clothes

Take enough clothes for the baby to wear for at least four days. Work on about two outfits per day, as you'll have to change your baby's clothes more often in case of spit-ups. Even though some super cute outfits are available in the shops, pack something comfortable instead. Soft onesies are always a good option.

Socks and beanies

As we've mentioned, newborns can't generate their own body heat due to their limited body fat and their little body's inability to metabolize the fat. They also can't shiver, a way in which a person can increase body heat. Make sure your baby will be warm enough. Even if your baby's onesie covers their feet, put a pair of socks on their tiny feet underneath the outfit. Babies lose a lot of their body heat through their heads, so pack at least one beanie to wear daily.

Blankets

Take some receiving and warm blankets. Receiving blankets are great to use to swaddle a baby. Warm blankets can be great when you do skin-to-skin contact since your baby will only wear a diaper, and you won't have your shirt on during this time. Make sure you both stay warm.

Diapers

Some hospitals will provide diapers for your baby's stay, while others request you to bring them. Make sure to find out the policy for the hospital your partner will be giving birth. If ever in doubt, pack a couple of diapers in the bag, and leave more in the car or with someone you know will be there as soon as visitors are allowed.

Wet wipes

The same goes for wet wipes. Some hospitals will provide them, while others expect you to bring enough for your stay. If you need to take your own supply, don't think one packet will be enough. Especially while the baby's passing meconium, the baby's first dark and extremely sticky poos. You might use a whole box of wipes on a single diaper change.

Creams

Here's a good tip to impress your wife with about meconium. Put some petroleum jelly on your baby's bum after every diaper change. The meconium will then stick to the Vaseline, not your baby's skin, making these diapers extremely easy and quick to change. Otherwise, remember to pack some bum cream to protect your baby's sensitive skin.

Toiletries

If you need to take toiletries for your baby, remember to pack body wash, body lotion, cotton balls, and surgical spirits or rubbing alcohol for cleaning the umbilical cord. Make sure all the toiletries you get for your baby are for sensitive skin. Many newborns' skins struggle with heavily fragranced products.

Burp cloth

Make sure your partner has a burp cloth ready every time she feeds or burps the baby. This can help to prevent milk spills on your clothes. We will discuss this in more detail in Chapter 8.

Pacifiers

If you decide to use a pacifier for your baby, make sure to pack that, as well as a small microwave sterilizer to clean them at the hospital. There are many benefits to using a pacifier, such as soothing a crying baby and preventing sudden infant death syndrome.

When to Go to the Hospital

It's important to know when it's time to rush your wife to the hospital when she's in labor. We've discussed the difference between Braxton Hicks contractions and true labor, so you should be able to tell when actual labor is starting. However, contractions can continue for a good couple of hours before active labor starts. The longer you can keep your partner comfortable at home, the easier the process will be for both of you.

Your wife's OB-GYN will advise you when you must go to the hospital, and many follow the popular 5-1-1 rule. According to this, you should head to the hospital once your wife's contractions are five minutes apart, last for one minute, and continue for one hour. Keep in mind that your wife's individual case might cause your OB-GYN to advise differently, so always follow the doctor's advice.

If your wife experiences any signs of actual labor starting before she reaches 37 weeks, or if she has any vaginal bleeding, extreme dizziness, or blurred vision, take her to the hospital immediately. These can all be signs of complications, and your OB-GYN will need to examine and possibly treat your wife.

Premature Birth

If your baby's born before 37 weeks of pregnancy, it'll be classified as premature birth. It's divided into four categories (Mayo Clinic, 2021):

- **Late preterm** is when the baby's born between 34 and 36 weeks of pregnancy.
- **Moderately preterm** is when the baby's born between 32 and 34 weeks of pregnancy.
- **Very preterm** is when the baby's born earlier than 32 weeks of pregnancy.
- **Extreme preterm** is when the baby's born earlier than 25 weeks of pregnancy.

These babies can have an increased risk of medical and developmental issues, and since some of the major organs, particularly their lungs, won't be fully developed yet, they will likely spend at least a couple of weeks in the neonatal intensive care unit (NICU) at the hospital.

Apart from breathing difficulties, your baby might need help with feeding, as they may not have developed the ability to suck or swallow yet. This will then be done by inserting a feeding tube through their noses. The baby's gastrointestinal system might not have matured yet, which can lead to conditions such as necrotizing enterocolitis, where the lining of the bowel wall is injured. As scary as this can be, trust your baby's doctors. As parents, there isn't much you can do to relieve any swelling or discomfort your baby might experience.

Babies born prematurely also have an increased risk of suffering from anemia, jaundice, immune disorders, bleeding in the brain (intraventricular hemorrhage), and heart conditions such as patent ductus arteriosus, where there's an opening between the pulmonary artery and aorta.

Premature birth can lead to serious long-term complications, including cerebral palsy, problems with learning, hearing and vision issues, chronic health problems, and behavioral and psychological difficulties.

As much as it's good to take note of the problems that can arise from premature birth, don't dwell too much on this. Should your wife go into premature labor, your OB-GYN will do everything possible to stop the labor. If these steps are unsuccessful and your baby's born prematurely, specialists such as neonatologists and pediatricians will care for your little one and try to reduce any risk of serious complications. Increasing your knowledge of all the possibilities of what might happen will give you the confidence to deal with these potential situations.

Let's Talk About Birth

Contractions are one of the most obvious signs of labor, but there are many other signs of labor starting that you can look out for. One of the first signs is a change in vaginal discharge, followed by a mucus plug or bloody show. This can be a pinkish or even brown jelly-like discharge, indicating the opening of her cervix. This doesn't necessarily mean labor is starting but normally indicates that labor is usually a couple of days away. Don't freak out when your wife shows you her bloody show. It'll likely not put you off eating Jell-O forever.

She might suddenly get the urge to go to the bathroom. This is caused by the baby's head pushing on her bowels. Without going into too much information here, having good bowel movements early on in labor can help your wife feel a lot more comfortable during labor. When she gets to the point of pushing the baby out, she pushes in the same way she would normally during a bowel movement. This often causes the pregnant woman to poop on the delivery table. If this happens to your wife, she might be embarrassed afterward. Don't make a big deal of it. Your OB-GYN or the nursing staff will quickly wipe the poo away. This is normal. If the doctor or nurse can deal with it without making a face, so can you.

An obvious sign that she's in labor will be when your partner's water breaks. This happens when the amniotic sac breaks, and amniotic fluid leaks out through her vagina. There's usually not much doubt when your wife's water breaks. However, don't ever wait for her water to break if her contractions meet the 5-1-1 rule. In many cases, the amniotic sac doesn't break naturally, and your OB-GYN will have to break it using a long plastic hook. Should this happen to your wife, stay calm. It shouldn't be painful for her; even if it is, it'll be nothing compared to the contractions she's experiencing. Once your partner's water breaks, your baby will most likely have to be delivered within 24 hours.

Can You Be in the Delivery Room?

If you've ever wondered whether you should be in the delivery room for your baby's birth, stop having those thoughts right now. Your wife will need you there, even if it's just to calm her or so she can have a hand to squash during delivery. You'll also not want to miss your baby being born. However, some women do prefer their partners not to be there. Have a conversation with your wife about this beforehand, so you'll both know what the expectations are.

There are some general guidelines to be aware of the minute you step into the delivery room. The main reason you're there is to support your partner. Yes, you also want to experience your baby's birth. You'll be the least important person in the room. This is about your wife and the baby.

In the same way, as it's good to find out if your partner wants you in the delivery room, it can be helpful to discuss expectations before your wife goes into labor. Find out if she wants you to take photos or videos during delivery. Maybe all she wants is for you to hold her hand or help her with deep breathing. Either way, you'll earn some brownie points by being considerate enough to ask.

Keep your own limitations in mind when discussing these expectations. If you easily get queasy or squeamish by the sight of blood, don't volunteer to be front and center. Tell your wife you'd prefer to stand by her head and support her from there. Don't force yourself to do something you're not comfortable with.

Whatever you do, be the support she needs. Also, be aware that she might not be in a position to tell you what you can do to help her. If you took childbirth classes, try the tips given there. Otherwise, try different things to help her. Unless her doctor advises against it, you can offer her ice chips. You might think giving her a back rub will help her to deal with the pain. Yes, this might help, or it might not. If your wife screams at you to stop, then stop, smile, and try something else. Remember, she's birthing a child right now, so maybe give her space and grace to yell. Just support her! She's dealing with a lot of pain, so try anything. Trying is better than standing around being in the way. Chances are, if you do nothing to help, you'll also get shouted at. So, rather do something than nothing.

Despite what you might feel at the moment, wondering what you can do to help her is the easy part of the job. Labor is anything but easy. Regardless of how difficult it can be seeing your wife in severe pain and not knowing what to do to help her, her job of delivering the baby's a lot more difficult. Guys, you might feel like you'll die while you have the man flu. Believe me, man-flu is nothing like childbirth. Many medical professionals compare the pain from labor to breaking 20 bones in your body simultaneously. It isn't a pain you can truly explain to others. And it'll just get worse and worse until the minute the baby's shoulders are out. Be her advocate and make sure all her needs are met. This will help her focus only on giving birth without worrying about anything else.

Never focus on the clock in the delivery room. As much as it's essential to time her contractions before going to the hospital, you should forget any reference to time once you're there. The nursing staff will make sure the labor progresses. If your partner ever asks you how long the labor has been, try to be as vague as possible. Knowing that she has been at it for 19 hours won't motivate her or put her in a positive mindset. Instead, answer her something like this, "It's been a while, but we're getting there."

Always stay calm. You might see things that you wish you could unsee. Man up. It's part of this process. Never ever say anything is "gross" or 'disgusting." Don't react negatively when the family drives you insane by asking for updates. They are just as excited as you about adding this little human to the family. It can be helpful to create a group chat to add everyone who might want an update. Better yet, set the group so you can only send a message to it. And then, put your phone on silent if you still receive too many requests for updates. Your calmness will make her calmer.

This ties in with the next important point: Don't spend unnecessary time on your phone once you're in the delivery room. Make sure you show her that you're connected, committed, and with her every step of the way.

When she's crying or cursing from pain, don't tell her anything along the lines of, "It can't be that bad." Fellas, it is that bad and worse. Also, never compare it to any pain you ever might have had. That time you bumped your pinkie toe against the leg of the coffee table was nothing compared to what she's going through. Just hold her hand (or rather, allow her to squash the life out of it) or her leg, and if you have to talk, tell her how great she's doing or how proud of her you are.

Lastly, don't become a backseat pusher when it's time to push this new life out. The OB-GYN, midwife, or nurse will tell your wife what to do when to push, and when not to push. If you also get involved, it can become like a sporting event, with your yelling "push" getting louder and louder. Rather stay quiet, let her squeeze the life out of your hand, and encourage her in a low and calm tone when necessary.

Pain Management During Labor

Pain management should be discussed with your OB-GYN in the weeks leading up to labor. Many women opt to go for non-medical pain relief options, with many changing their minds mid-labor when the true effects of contractions can be felt. It often happens that when the mom-to-be changes her mind, her labor can have progressed too far, and she'll have no other option but to (literally!) push through. This is why it's important to know all her options before going into labor.

Let's first discuss the non-medical methods of relieving labor pains:

Antenatal or birthing classes

These can help a pregnant woman know what to expect, reducing the anxiety of childbirth. Many medical professionals argue that if you know what to expect, you can deal with pain and other uncomfortableness easier. Another way to reduce her anxiety and, as a result, help her deal with the pain is to have her partner (yes, that's you!) with her to support her.

Being fit and healthy

This is another way that can help a woman deal with labor, as she will generally have more energy and endurance. This is why it's so important to moderate exercise for as long as possible during pregnancy.

Deep breathing techniques

Many methods are known to help women get through contractions. Your wife will learn these techniques during birthing classes. Your OB-GYN, midwife, or nurse will also help your wife with her breathing during labor.

Using music

This can be a welcoming distraction that can help her deal with the pain of labor, but if she's against this, please turn it off immediately. Jamming to

"Gangnam Style" might not be her cup of tea right now.

A massage

This can look like using oil, hot or cold packs, and a warm shower. If there's a handheld shower-head, she can use this to apply hot water straight to her tummy or lower back. Should she decide to shower during labor, prioritize staying close to the bathroom in case she needs help. Although these natural techniques can help, many women don't find them effective enough to relieve their labor pain. Although other medical methods can be used to reduce the feeling of pain, the following are the most popular choices used worldwide:

Nitrous oxide

If you've ever seen a pregnant woman in a movie yell, "Give me the gas!" this is what she was referring to. This gas is administered through a face mask whenever she has a contraction. This method doesn't take the pain away but takes the edge off and distracts the laboring woman as she's concentrating on inhaling the gas. Nitrous oxide doesn't affect the baby but can cause possible mild side effects for the mom-to-be, including nausea and vomiting, confusion, and disorientation.

Pethidine

This pain reliever is in a similar class as morphine and is administered by injection. Its impact can last up to four hours and can effectively relieve labor pains. Possible side effects for mom include nausea and vomiting, disorientation, and slower breathing. It can also affect the unborn baby's breathing and ability to suck after birth. If this is the case, your doctor will administer a reversal drug for your baby. In most cases, however, the effects of the pethidine will have worked out before your baby's born.

Epidural

This is the most effective form of pain relief during labor. An anesthetic is injected into the mom-to-be's spinal cord, making her feel numb from the waist down. After getting an epidural, the OB-GYN will monitor the unborn baby's heart rate closely to make sure the baby doesn't go into fetal distress. Possible side effects include feeling faint and nauseated. A urinary catheter will have to be inserted, as she will have no bladder control, headaches, and muscle weakness in the legs, which can last for an hour or more after your baby's born. It can also affect the pregnant woman's ability to push during labor, resulting in a vacuum cup or forceps being used to deliver the baby.

What's a C-Section?

Complications can arise that will make a vaginal birth either too dangerous or even impossible. Usually, this will be called weeks ahead of time, but something can also happen during vaginal delivery, causing the OB-GYN to change the birthing plan. In cases like this, a C-section will be done to surgically remove the baby from the pregnant woman's uterus.

If this does happen to your wife, don't stress or freak out. About 30% of all babies in the United States are born via C-section (WebMD, n.d.). This form of birth is generally perfectly safe for both mom and baby, but since it's a major surgery where the doctor will cut through many layers of ligaments and muscles in the mom's tummy, it can make caring for the newborn more difficult. Your partner will have postoperative pain and won't be able to bend down or pick up anything heavy. Time to show your new daddy superpowers!

An epidural or spinal block will be administered before the operation, numbing the pregnant woman from the waist down. This means she'll be awake during the surgery and can see her baby minutes, if not seconds, after the baby's removed from the uterus. A screen is placed between the woman's head and body to ensure she can't see the actual operation. Without serious complications, the dad-to-be can be in the operating room during this procedure. You'll sit by your wife's head. Again, if you're squeamish at all, look at her face and not the operation. You don't want to cause a commotion by fainting midway through the birth of your baby. The whole procedure only takes between 30 to 45 minutes.

Many complications can make a C-section the safest form of delivery. If the following happens, your OB-GYN will likely perform a planned C-section:

- the baby being breech (feet to the bottom, head up) or traverse (sideways)
- the baby has congenital disabilities detected on an ultrasound scan, such as hydrocephalus
- the baby's too big to fit through the birth canal
- placenta previa (when the placenta is very low in the uterus or covers the cervix)
- multiple births
- the mother had a previous C-section or any form of operation on her uterus

As we've mentioned, a C-section can be performed if complications arise during labor:

- labor stops midway through
- the baby's in fetal distress
- placenta abruption (when the placenta separates from the uterine wall)
- the umbilical cord is tight around the baby's neck
- the umbilical cord enters the birth canal before the baby

There you go... You just learned a lot of information to impress your wife (and possibly even your OB-GYN). You'll now not only be able to reassure your wife with the statistics on how common C-sections are but will even be able to list the reasons for needing a C-section. You'll be able to stay calm and keep your partner calm. Brownie points are coming your way!

Checking Baby's Health

Shortly after your baby's born, a doctor will examine your little one. If the baby's born full-term, the specialist will be called a pediatrician. Should your baby be preterm, a neonatologist or a pediatrician will look after your baby's health.

If the delivery takes place via a C-section, this specialist will be in the operating room from the beginning of the procedure. This is because C-section babies often struggle to start breathing, as their breathing isn't stimulated to start naturally by moving through the birth canal. If this is the case with your baby, the pediatrician will replicate this stimulation to get the breathing going. If this happens, don't freak out. Pediatricians are trained to do this and probably help hundreds (if not more) of babies every year to start breathing. Stand by your wife, act as if everything is going perfectly, and wait for those first cries.

The sound of your baby's first cries might surprise you. It doesn't sound anything like the overwhelming cry you might get used to in just a couple of weeks. Those first cries actually sound more like a cat crying than a tiny human. Take this in, or better yet, make a video of your newborn's cat cries. Within only a couple of hours, this will be gone, and the crying will sound normal—a sound you'll get used to over the next couple of months.

The doctor or nursing staff will also perform two Apgar tests on your baby. This is a quick, non-invasive test done first a minute after birth to evaluate how the baby handled the birthing process and again after five minutes, to assess how the baby's coping after birth. On rare occasions, this test may be repeated again after 10 minutes. This test looks at five aspects: color, heart rate, reflexes, muscle tone, and breathing. A score of either zero, one, or two is given for each element, making up a score out of ten. The higher the score, the better your baby's coping.

Practical New Dad Tip

Discuss getting help before your child comes. Knowing who you have in your corner to support you during this new chapter is a great way to have peace of mind. Whether that is family helping out, friends, or hired help, it's great to have the discussion so you're aware of what you have available in any situation you might find yourself in. You might also need someone to fetch things from home that you've either forgotten or didn't think of packing. The saying goes, "It takes a village to raise a child" (Dubner, 2011). Find your village and accept their offers of help.

7

NATIONAL CHAMPION

You now have the most treasured prize of all! You and your partner have brought a child into this world. Congratulations! This is even better than being a state champion. In fact, you've created your own little national champion!

You've now reached what many people call the fourth trimester of pregnancy. Your baby has been born, but now it's time to step up your dad game. Your life has changed forever for the better. Having a newborn in the home can be challenging, and many dads would prefer to fast forward through the coming months to when their child is old enough to interact and kick a ball with them. Don't be *that* dad.

As much as you can look forward to having your own homegrown teammate, enjoy these coming months (even though it can be exhausting) and bond with your little one as much as you can.

You Have a Child, Now What?

After you've fulfilled one of your first duties of taking as many photos as possible and ensuring your wife settles into the maternity ward and gets some bonding time, it's now time for you to become a gate-keeper. The minute you let people know you're officially a dad, they will likely ask what time the hospital's visiting hours are or even just rock up there unannounced.

Your partner might be exhausted after delivery, and as much as she's looking forward to showing off your bundle of joy, both of you need to have a couple of moments to reflect on what happened, take it all in, and spend time with the baby. Your job is to support your wife and make sure she's as comfortable as possible.

If you don't feel up to having visitors yet, don't be afraid to tell them that you'll let them know when they can visit. If they arrive at the hospital uninvited, explain to them that you need time alone with the baby or that your wife is too tired. They will probably be so excited to see the baby that they won't mind waiting at the hospital's coffee shop or coming back later once all three of you are ready for people.

Once you start letting in visitors, confirm they wash their hands thoroughly as they enter the room. If anyone is sick—even the slightest sniffs—ask them to rather stay outside. Your baby will still need to build its little immune system, and the last thing you want is for your newborn to get sick (although this happens more often than you might realize). Never let anyone kiss your baby on the mouth or even on the hands. Remember, babies often put their hands in their mouths when they get hungry.

The hospital's visitation policy will likely stipulate this but never allow too many visitors simultaneously. Apart from potentially exposing your baby to germs, your little one can also get overstimulated by all the different faces, voices, and smells, and their bodies can get sore from being held like that. Protect your baby better than you would an NFL Super Bowl ring.

Breastfeeding

Most medical professionals will encourage your partner to breastfeed your baby. Breastmilk holds numerous benefits for the baby: It's filled with the vitamins and minerals your baby will need, is highly nutritious, offers protection against some infections, and can reduce the risk of sudden infant death syndrome, the unexplained death of a baby younger than one-year-old.

Depending on how she gave birth, the nurses will put the baby on her breast as soon as possible after birth, usually within only a few minutes. This first attempt is often unsuccessful, as your wife and baby will still be recovering from the beautiful trauma they just experienced. Babies generally don't need to feed for about an hour after birth, so if the first time doesn't work, she can try nursing again later. The nursing staff will help your wife and baby get the perfect latch. If there are problems, they will check your baby's blood sugar regularly to assess that it doesn't drop too low due to not getting any (or enough) milk. If this does happen, they will give the baby little bits of formula (often using a cup to not cause any nipple confusion) to take the edge off their hunger. If your wife continues to struggle, consider arranging a consultation with a lactation specialist in your area. The staff at the maternity ward, OB-GYN, or pediatrician will be able to recommend one. Alternatively, a quick online search will give you a list of specialists to consider.

Newborn babies must feed every two to three hours, give or take. For at least the first six weeks, or until the pediatrician gives the okay, it's important to wake your baby up for feeds. If they skip a feed, their blood sugar can drop very quickly to dangerously low levels. If your baby wants to feed more frequently than that, don't starve them. Feed them on demand when they are hungry. Apart from crying, signs that a newborn wants to feed include the following:

- Smacking their lips.
- Sticking their tongues out.
- Searching with their heads for a nipple (especially when you hold them close to you).
- Sucking their hands.

Since your partner will spend more than half a day breastfeeding your baby, it can be exhausting. Your wife will appreciate every bit of help, no matter how small it may seem. Be an extra set of hands for her. Your partner will need this, as breastfeeding will take over her entire life for a bit. Help her clean the breast pump's different parts after each use, or get an extra golden star by baking her lactation cookies to snack on. Many recipes are available online and are so easy to make that they are relatively foolproof.

Even though you won't be able to physically help with the middle-of-the-night feeds, there are many ways you can make these feeds easier on her. Get up to change the diaper, or burp the baby once the feed is done. This way, your wife can get some more rest. If you're afraid to burp the baby or don't know how to do this (after all, your burps come out naturally by themselves), don't fret, we'll discuss this and give helpful tips in Chapter 8.

Apart from supporting her with logistics, be there for her emotionally. Many women can't breastfeed. This can be due to having inverted nipples or insufficient glandular breast tissue to produce sufficient milk. Others have to stop due to allergies or illness. This can wreak a mama emotionally, making her feel like the worst mother for not being able to feed her baby. Be a rock for your wife. Remind her to stop feeling guilty. There are brilliant formulas on the market.

In the end, the only thing that truly matters is that your baby's fed. Choose the method—breastfeeding, expressing (when mom pumps and provides the breast milk with a bottle), or using formula—that fits into your life. In a couple of years, your child will likely eat old French fries off a dirty carpet in the car, so ultimately, whether a child is breast- or bottle-fed isn't a life-or-death decision. Just make sure your baby isn't hungry.

If she does breastfeed, remember that mama's boobs are now holding your baby's food. Should your wife allow you some playtime there and you do get a mouthful of milk, don't freak out. Swallow it as quickly as possible without mentioning it or spit it out. Remember that if you make a big deal out of it, you might not be allowed close to them again, so choose your best option carefully.

Your Family Is Home

Just as you and your partner seem to settle into your roles as parents (with the help of the nursing staff, of course), you hear the most surprisingly frightening words: Mom and baby have been discharged. It's now time to put on your big boy undies. You're about to take an actual living baby home. You and your partner will be solely responsible for keeping your baby alive. If a profanity or two slips out, no one will blame you. This can be scary. Remember the tip on practicing how to use the baby seat for the car? You're probably thanking me right about now...

Once you're home, take as much off her plate as possible. She'll be exhausted, and her body will need time to recover. If you have time off from work (paternity leave), let her rest as much as possible. Look after your baby (especially during the first two weeks they will sleep most of the time), do the laundry, wash the dishes, clean the house, and cook food. Some of your loved ones might offer to bring meals. Even if you don't like a specific aunt's cooking, accept it with a smile. It's one less thing for you and your partner to worry about.

You might notice your newborn's skin gets a yellowish tinge after a few days. This is jaundice and is a surprisingly common occurrence in newborns. The best home remedy for this is to expose the baby's skin (through a window or lace curtain) to sunlight daily. Use this as an excuse to relax and bond with the baby. Sit in a comfy chair, and let your baby sleep on your chest. If you want to be a super dad, remove your shirt and combine it with skin-to-skin contact. You will be a miracle jaundice healer, your wife will also have some time to relax, and your baby (and you) can have the first of many naps together.

While we're on the subject of skin-to-skin contact, you might wonder what the big deal of doing this is and even how to do this. Let's get into the how first: You simply take off your shirt, take off the baby's clothes (but keep the diaper on!), and sit comfortably on a chair while you let your baby lay tummy down on your bare chest. Remember to cover your baby's back with a blanket to stay warm. Doing this holds endless benefits for your baby. Amongst others, it helps regulate your baby's heart rate and breathing, reduces the cortisol levels of both you and the baby, and provides a great bonding opportunity.

Another way to bond with your baby and help your wife is to take care of bath time. No boobs are needed to bathe a baby, so this is a sure way dad can help. Before they are discharged from the hospital, a nurse will likely give your baby their first bath. Go with them for this bath and take note of what the nurse is doing. If you follow these steps, bath time is easy. In fact, as long as you try your best to not get water in your baby's ears or let them drown, you can't go wrong here.

You might find yourself freaking out about nothing. If your baby sneezes, it might feel to you like they have pneumonia. You're not a hypochondriac. You're a new parent who wants the best for their little human. If you ever feel unsure, call your baby's pediatrician for advice. Remember, something that doesn't seem very serious with an infant can become life-threatening in a matter of hours. You'd rather call them unnecessarily than ignore something that could potentially be a serious concern. If any of the following happens, you should definitely make the call or take the baby to see the doctor (Ben-Joseph, 2018):

- rectal temperature of 100.4 °F (38 °C) in babies younger than two months
- bloody vomit or poo
- more than eight runny poos in eight hours (yes, your baby's poo won't only be of huge interest to you but also become a topic of conversation)
- fontanelle (soft spot on your baby's head) bulging out
- fast breathing, particularly if your baby turns blue around the mouth
- difficulty waking your baby up
- signs of dehydration
- sunken eyes
- no wet diapers for six hours
- crying without tears
- fontanelle sinking in

Your Life Has Changed

If your work permits time off as paternity leave, take it. Even if you don't feel like you need it, it's essential to spend this time at home, bonding with your baby and helping your partner adjust to her new role as a mom... and yours as a first-time dad!

You'll both be sleep-deprived, and chances are this will continue for at least a couple of weeks. On top of this, you'll be nervous about ensuring your newborn's needs are met and may also feel anxious about this journey.

While your wife and baby will be your top priorities, it's crucial that you still make time for yourself. Make time to do something you enjoy, even if it's just a quick stop at the gym on the way home from work or reading an extra comic book while sitting on the toilet. Give your wife the same opportunity to do something by herself. If she's breastfeeding, this will have to be between feeds. Make sure you're there for her.

Self-care is vital in this new phase of your life. If you deplete all your energy, it'll have a significant impact on your new family. Do what you need to do to make sure you stay sane. Look out for any signs of post-partum depression in yourself and your partner. Support each other and, if need be, seek professional help. Your baby needs their parents mentally strong to take care of them.

Practical New Dad Tip

Wet wipes are the Swiss Army knife for babies and toddlers. Have extra sets of baby wipes in all places of your home and living space. Place them in the living room, bedroom, kitchen, backyard, and car, and make sure there are always tons of wipes in the diaper bag. You never know when you'll need them. Your partner will forever be grateful for planning ahead.

TIME TO BE A DAD

N ow that you're a father and have brought your brand new family member home, it's time for you to be a dad. You've made it through the pregnancy, you (and your partner) have survived the birth, your hand has recovered from being squeezed during labor, and all three of you have settled back home.

The worst part is over. However, you might still feel unsure about how to care for your baby. As fragile as they look (and are), they don't break easily. Get those fears of picking your tiny human up out of your mind. Otherwise, you'll never get to bond with your little one or help your wife with parenting duties.

Let's get the first thing out of the way. When you're looking after your child, never call it babysitting. A babysitter is someone you pay to look after your child when you're not available. Unless you're getting paid for looking after your child, you're not babysitting. You're parenting and being a father, not just a sperm donor who helped to create the baby and can now sit back and relax.

You're Officially a Parent

Being a dad doesn't mean you'll chill on the couch while your wife does all the nursing, caring, and bonding. Being a dad means being involved, from changing those soiled diapers to burping your baby and calming them when they cry.

Don't run for the hills now. As overwhelming as this might sound, being a dad will soon be second nature, especially if you use these handy tips.

Handling Your Baby

Always supporting the baby's neck is the most important thing to remember when handling and holding your newborn. Very young babies have weak neck muscles and can't hold their heads (which might seem way too big for their little bodies) up by themselves. If you pick a young baby up without supporting their neck, you might cause their head to dangle or flop, which could cause not only damage to their fragile neck but also severe brain injury. When you pick your new baby up, always place one hand under the baby's neck and support the lower back or bum with your other hand or arm. As long as you do this, your baby will be fine. You can do this! At first, you might concentrate that your hands are in the right place, but after doing this a couple of times, it'll feel completely natural. You'll even be able to do this half-asleep during a night-time feed.

Continue supporting your baby's neck until its muscles are strong enough to hold its head up by themselves. This usually happens between three to six months. Don't "test" the strength of your baby's neck by removing the support. Instead, keep an eye on your baby when they are enjoying tummy time or lying down. Once you see them lifting their heads by themselves, you'll know you can start to slowly reduce the support.

Change a Diaper

Changing a baby's diaper is probably one of the worst jobs as a parent, but if you want a happy marriage, don't expect your wife to do this task alone. Mentally prepare yourself for this, as you'll do this often because babies can be pooping machines. It's easy to determine if your baby needs a change. If the diaper is filled with wee, it'll feel full and heavy, while you'll be able to smell a poop diaper, sometimes a mile away.

If you do get the whiff, make sure you have plenty of wet wipes close to you before you start removing the baby's clothes. Alternatively, get the bath water ready. Babies can leave waste explosions at times that won't only need almost a whole packet of wipes to clean, but a bath might also be necessary to make sure no excess poop is left on the skin. The acidity in their poop can irritate or burn a baby's sensitive skin very quickly.

To determine the level of hazard you're dealing with, you can gently pull the diaper away from the baby's back or thigh and have a quick peek. This can also help you determine whether you should grab a gas mask to protect yourself from the violent smell that can feel like a bullet to the head once it hits you.

Once you know what you're dealing with, get all the necessary equipment ready. Apart from the gas mask, bath water, and wipes, this will also include a clean diaper, bum cream to protect the sensitive skin against irritation by the excretions, and sometimes even a clean set of clothes in the case of a severe explosion.

If you have a boy, always put a wet wipe, face cloth, or another sort of cover over the penis during diaper changes. If not, you risk getting hit in the face by a tiny pee fountain. Also, point the penis down when putting on a new diaper. Otherwise, you'll end up changing your little peeing machine's clothes more often than his diapers.

When putting on a new diaper, always remember the side with the sticky tabs on is the back. The sticky tabs fasten on the front of the diaper. You should secure the diaper enough to stay in position but never too tight. You can do a quick finger test to determine if it's too tight: If you can slide your finger between your baby's skin and diaper with relative ease, it should be fine. Once you're done and the baby's clothed, pat yourself on the back.

Burp Your Baby

In the first three months of a baby's life, it's important to burp them after every feed, sometimes even in the middle of one. This is because babies swallow a lot of air bubbles as they drink, which will cause discomfort for the baby afterward. Imagine yourself downing a gallon of beer and the discomfort the gassiness will cause. This is similar to what a baby feels. Only their little bodies can't burp (or sometimes even fart) by themselves.

There are many ways to burp a baby. One of the most common methods is to let your baby sit on your lap and support their neck by placing one hand under their chin. Gently rub your baby's back, bottom to top, repeatedly. You can also bounce your leg, but make sure these are minimal movements. You don't want to shake your baby doing this. You can also let your baby lie stomach down over your lap, with their belly resting on your thigh, or hold your baby against your chest with their chin resting on your shoulder. Rub your baby's back from the bottom to the top, or pat your baby's back gently.

Make sure you always have a burp cloth ready, as a baby often spits up a bit of milk as they burp. Let me give you a little warning: Don't wear your newest work shirt when doing this. These gentle burps can sometimes turn into projectile vomiting, which can not only stain your shirt but leave you smelling just as sour as your mood might be.

Calm Your Crying, Baby

Knowing how to comfort your baby when they cry can go a long way in preserving your sanity. Some babies cry more than others, seemingly for no reason whatsoever. If this is the case for you, the word "colic" will probably start feeling like profanity. Colic happens when your crying machine revs up at specific times of the day, sometimes for hours at a time, with no apparent reason or cause for the crying.

Unfortunately, no matter how healthy the mom's pregnancy is or how smoothly the birth goes, there's no way to know if your baby will be crabby or happy. It's the luck of the draw. If your baby does have colic, this usually subsides after three to six months. During this time, remember those grandmas, grandpas, aunts, and uncles who will be eager to look after your scream machine while you and your wife recharge outside the house.

If you want to be a super dad in a happy marriage, here is a checklist of what you can look out for when your baby cries:

Diaper

Do a quick smell and feel test. You'd also cry if you pooped your pants and were left to lay in the poop. Remember, the diaper doesn't have to be soiled to bother your baby. A soggy diaper is heavy and restricts a baby's movement.

Hungry

If it's almost time for a feed, get the bottle ready or hand the baby over to mom for some boob recharge. While your wife's breastfeeding your baby, pretend you need to do something urgently outside and go catch a breath of fresh air to decompress. Remember, it's important to take care of yourself too. I don't intend to sound like a broken record, but taking care of you is necessary. Then, rush back to burp the baby or catch and clean any projectile vomit.

Tired or overstimulated

Small babies are supposed to sleep most of the day. If the *crank o' meter* shoots up after your baby has been awake for a while, it might be tired or overstimulated. Keep in mind that your baby had little to no excitement in the womb, so seeing the world might get a bit much for them. Take them to a quiet room to relax and fall asleep.

Too hot or cold

Young babies can't regulate their body heat yet, so you'll always need to dress them correctly. The general rule of thumb is to dress your baby in one more layer than you're wearing.

Gas

If your crying machine revs up shortly after a feed, try to burp your baby again. If burping doesn't help, your baby might struggle to fart (yes, that does happen). Lay them on their back and move their legs up and down like they are riding a bicycle, or massage their stomach in a clockwise, circular movement.

Lonely

If your baby wakes up screaming alone in the crib in the room, they might want someone to hold them and make them feel safe and secure. Get your bonding going by cuddling with your little one.

Sick

Unfortunately, babies are born with no immune system to protect them from germs, so they get sick easily. Do yourself a favor and invest in a forehead thermometer. Check their temperatures if you find no other source for the extra crabbiness. If that seems fine, see if their noses are congested or gently push on the tragus (the triangular piece of ear covering the opening) of their ears. If your baby has an earache, their crying will turn to screaming from touching the ear. Now you know it's time to visit the doctor. If their noses are congested, you use a couple of drops of saline nasal spray or breastmilk to loosen the snot. Also, consider investing in a little device you use to suck the snot from your baby's nose. It sounds disgusting, but trust me, the relief your baby will experience will make life much more pleasant for everyone around. And these devices do have little sponges in to make sure no snot will get to your mouth while sucking. It'll be fine!

If you've ticked everything on your checklist and your baby's still a cranky pant, don't lose hope. Try the following five things before you order noise-canceling earphones:

Pacifier

Not all babies like to suckle on a pacifier, but it can do wonders to keep the crying machine quiet. Some people are against the use of a pacifier, as it can spread germs if the pacifier falls on the ground, can cause a couple of sleepless nights when you want to take it away, and if you don't and let your baby use it for too long, it can cause problems with speech development and the forming of their mouth, which can result in crooked teeth. Talk to your partner and decide if you want to use one.

Swaddle

In the womb, babies don't have a lot of room for movement, which is why they often calm down when wrapped tightly in blankets.

Let them swing. Many parents swear by using a motorized swing. This calms the baby, as the movement is similar to what they felt in mom's womb when she was walking (or waddling closer to the end).

White noise

While in the womb, your baby constantly hears noises similar to white noise. This is why the sound of a vacuum cleaner, dishwasher, or washing machine can be so comforting for a baby. Doing the laundry can score you a double whammy of brownie points.

Put them in the car

This has proven to be highly effective when soothing a baby. Strap them into their car seat, leave mom at home to enjoy some quiet time, and go for a drive. If it's close to dinner time, go past a drive-through restaurant and pick up something for supper— kudos for your incredible thinking right there!

Bonding With Your Child

After carrying the baby for nine months, giving birth to them, and then caring for them, your wife will already have a special bond with your little one. Since she'll likely be home on maternity leave, she'll also have more than enough time alone with the baby to cuddle and get to know their little quirks, likes, and dislikes.

This might not come as quickly for you, as you may only be home for a couple of days if you're lucky and won't have that automatic bonding that something like breastfeeding brings. You'll have to consciously work towards getting to know your tiny human. The best way to do this is to spend as much time with your baby as possible. Remember that quality is always more important than quantity, so even if you don't have much time to spend with your little one, make the most of what you have. The bond will come.

No matter how tired you might be after a long day at work and not sleeping properly since the baby's birth, you'll never have this time with your baby again. This sounds so cliché, I know, but it's the truth. Use every minute you can spare to bond with your little one. Before you know it, they will be teenagers with raging hormones, and you'll wish you had a sweet baby again.

As much as you want to sleep, getting up at night when your baby's fussy can be great for one-on-one bonding. They won't always want to drink when crying at night, often called the "witching hours." Sometimes, as we've mentioned, they will only want to be held and to feel secure. And, who better to make them feel safe than their superhero of a daddy? Soon, this little one will be your real-life sidekick, so set them up for this role now.

If your baby's wide awake at night and there doesn't seem to be much chance of getting them settled anytime soon, make the most of this time. Take the baby to the living room and put some sports highlights on the television. At some point during their lives, you'll have the opportunity to explain all the rules of your favorite sport to your little one. And there's no rule against starting this super early in their lives.

When you speak to your baby, try your best to always look them in the eyes. A newborn's eyesight isn't fully developed, so bring your face close to theirs...As long as you are not sick, of course! Let your baby touch your face and pull your scruff. They are learning all there is to know about their daddy. Sing to your baby. They don't care whether you can hold a note or not. All they want is to hear your voice. When spending time with them, echo their little sounds and mirror their facial expressions. Your baby's trying to communicate, and this is their only means at such an early stage of life.

You might soon realize that you enjoy this bonding time so much that you may want to do this as often as possible. Invest in a baby sling where you can carry your little one as you go about your duties at home. This will keep your baby close and connected to you, free up your hands to get things done and give mom a much-needed break.

If your partner starts expressing milk for bottle feeding, or if you decide to feed the baby formula, get involved in these feeds from the get-go. Initially, your baby might cry or be fussy when you try to feed them, as they are used to mom giving them milk. You might also feel unsure of what to do. Whatever you do, don't give up and simply hand the baby back to mom. The more you do it, the easier it'll become for both you and your baby.

Always remember that no matter how much you try, there's no such thing as a perfect parent. All parents make mistakes. It's part of life, and you will also make mistakes. As long as your baby's happy and kept alive, you're doing a great job. Congratulate yourself for being the best dad you can be, and try every day to be better than the last.

Babyproof Your Home

As your baby gets older and becomes more mobile, it's important to babyproof your home. One of the most important things to consider is making sure your electrical outlets are safe for your baby to be around. Various products on the market prevent your baby from sticking their little fingers in the outlets, jamming other things in there, or pulling a plug you're actively using. Go around your home and make notes of any electrical outlets in your baby's reach once they start crawling and walking. Make sure each one is covered.

You might think you don't need it, as you won't leave your baby unattended. However, trust me on this one. You have no idea how fast that little body can move. If you take your eyes off them for only a couple of seconds (while changing the channel on the television or checking a message on your phone), your baby might have moved to a danger zone, and you might just pull a muscle jumping up and running to keep them safe.

Also, look out for electrical wires that are hanging loose. Don't allow your baby to play tug of war with your television's cable. Chances are your baby will win the fight, with your television falling to pieces on the ground, possibly injuring your baby. You can get many cord rails or cable management boxes to reassure everything stays in place.

You can also look at different cabinets or magnetic locks to make sure your baby won't unpack your entire kitchen for you. These are particularly important for cupboards containing cleaning products or glassware. If you want to give your baby the chance to explore a little, you can leave your Tupperware cupboard unlocked. The baby won't harm themselves by unpacking this cupboard. Just look on the floor before entering the kitchen, as your baby might have turned your kitchen into a homemade obstacle course. You might harm yourself slipping on a plastic lid or board or trip over an empty cereal container stacked on top of another.

Once you're done with the electrical outlets and cables, look at anchoring your furniture. Many young children get seriously injured and can die from furniture falling onto them. For example, they don't understand the danger of pulling on a bookshelf and are more focused on discovering what is high on the bookshelf out of their reach. Children are natural climbers, and many can climb a bookshelf or chest of drawers before even walking properly. They will also use furniture to pull themselves up before standing up alone. You can use many brackets, wall mounts, and straps to anchor your furniture and appliances in position.

Regarding things you should put out of sight, don't leave any decorative items within your baby's reach, especially not glass or porcelain items that can break easily. Your friends and loved ones will know you used to have pretty things in your house, and they will understand why it has disappeared for now. Your baby's safety is much more important than having decorations in your home.

Another thing to consider is potted plants on the floors in your house. If your baby can reach them, they will likely dig out the soil in the pots, break off leaves, and even try to eat them. Remember that babies learn by putting things in their mouths. Many house plants are also poisonous if ingested, so removing this risk is always best by moving your potted plants out of reach.

Even loose throws and blankets can pose a risk. Your baby might get tangled in these, creating a risk of suffocation for young ones. Your cushions will likely also get scattered all over your lounge floor, so unless you want to pick them up daily, it might be a good idea to store them for the next couple of months.

Toilet seat clips are handy to keep little fingers out. Remember what we said above about babies putting things in their mouths to learn? Nothing that goes in the toilet should ever go in your baby's mouth, so rather keep it locked. Also, don't leave your toilet brush beside the toilet for easy access. The bristles of those brushes might feel great for itchy gums. I don't think we need to expand on why this is a horrible idea.

If you have stairs or a fireplace in your house, baby gates can be great for keeping your baby safe. Their muscles are still developing, and they shouldn't be climbing stairs alone. Slipping and tumbling down a staircase can happen so quickly.

Getting Lucky After Birth

Going through the first couple weeks of having a newborn, many men look forward to the six weeks mark. If your baby has gained healthy weight, your pediatrician might give you the good news that you can stop waking your baby up for night-time feeds. But that isn't all that happens at six weeks postpartum...

This is also when your wife will go for a postpartum checkup at her OB-GYN. Permitting no complications, the doctor might give your wife the all-clear for resuming intimacy.

If this is the case for your wife, it's excellent, as this means your wife's body has physically recovered from giving birth. However, don't ever pressure your wife to hop into bed. After everything she went through giving birth and having had to push a baby through her vajayjay, she might not feel emotionally or mentally ready to allow anything close to her lady again just yet.

She might fear getting pregnant again. This fear isn't unfounded. Many women, even those breastfeeding, can resume ovulation before reaching the six-week mark. This means that if you don't use contraceptives, she can get pregnant again. This can be something neither of you might be ready for. Her OB-GYN will likely discuss contraceptives with her and will probably give your partner a script for the contraceptive of her choice. If she chooses to use this, help her get her medication from the pharmacy. While you're there, get a packet of condoms. Depending on the type of contraceptive she'll use, it might take a couple of weeks to fully take effect. The condoms might make her feel more comfortable if there's double protection.

Also, grab a bottle or two of water-based lubrication while at the pharmacy. Due to her hormones still adjusting after giving birth, and especially if she's breastfeeding, she might experience vaginal dryness, which can make sex very painful. Using lube can help with this, plus a lot of foreplay to increase natural arousal.

Even with doing all of this, she might not agree to have sex just yet. If you're upset or irritated by this, don't show it to your wife. She has put her body through hell carrying your baby. Have patience with her, and try other forms of intimacy. Hold her hand, tell her how much you appreciate her, cuddle with her, kiss her, and if she allows, touch her. Build up to penetrative intimacy again. Take things as slowly as she needs them to be.

Once you eventually get the okay to raise your sails, she might experience pain. Ensure you have good communication, or look at her face for any signs of pain or discomfort. Although most women only feel pain during the first couple of times of penetration, for some, it can be painful for up to three months postpartum. If the pain persists, take her to see her OB-GYN. There might be a cause that can easily be treated.

Practical New Dad Tip

Find your village by joining Facebook groups about parenting or becoming a dad. These groups are great ways of staying connected with other new dads who are also going through this crazy, beautiful process for the first time. Having someone who understands what you're going through is beyond helpful.

CONCLUSION

You now have all the knowledge you need to rock being a first-time dad. You've also learned valuable facts to make this journey easier and impress your wife. Having gained all this insight on how to help your partner during the pregnancy and delivery, and caring for your little baby, already puts you one step ahead of most other dads-to-be or new dads.

You're now aware of everything that can possibly go wrong during a pregnancy and when to rush your partner to the doctor. Conversely, you'll know what seemingly weird or odd things can be perfectly normal. You also understand what you can do to make this pregnancy easier for your wife and what you need to consider when budgeting for your baby's care.

Most importantly, you understand that it's normal to doubt your abilities as a father and that the fears you might be feeling are common. Taking care of your and your partner's mental health will be a top priority, not only during pregnancy but also after the birth of your tiny human. On top of that, you know what you should and definitely shouldn't do during the birth of your baby, as well as how to care for your little one afterward.

You might feel like you've gone through information overload. That's okay. There's a lot to learn; luckily, you can go over the appropriate chapters as you experience that part of your journey. Let's recap some of the important things we've discussed to make things a bit easier for you.

You might deal with a lot of fears, such as being too selfish to be a good dad, loving your job or hanging out with the guys more than your baby, losing your identity, experiencing FOMO while having a newborn in the house, and even getting a "dad bod." These fears are normal. However, remember that your body was also made for being a dad, and the lowering of your testosterone levels shortly before your baby's due is scientific proof.

You might go through times during this journey when you feel your mental health declining. You might be worried about the many changes this pregnancy will bring to your life. Knowing what to expect and planning for it can help reduce your anxiety. Talk to your wife and create your birth plan. Remember to make four copies of this plan.

Have patience with your wife while she's pregnant. Her body will go through hell, starting from around week six of pregnancy and lasting all the way to the birth of your little one. Her boobs will get extremely sore and swollen. She might suffer from morning (or all-day) sickness. If she has weird cravings, just roll with it and buy her what she wants. Don't be sensitive to her mood swings. She can't help it. She may become forgetful. This strange phenomenon is called pregnancy brain. Help her through any difficulties in her pregnancy. Relieve her stress by giving a massage or making lists of what should be done.

If you want to impress your wife, plan a little getaway for the two of you before the baby's born. Go experience your babymoon! Find out what your wife would like to do, even if it's just relaxing in a hotel room with an air conditioner and room service.

Every pregnancy trimester comes with difficulties that your partner (and you) will go through. Important things that can happen during the first trimester include spotting, discharge, constipation, fatigue, frequent urination, and heartburn. Choose an OB-GYN to take care of your wife during the pregnancy and book an appointment. Get her a good prenatal vitamin. Get a healthy exercise routine going that you and your partner can do together. Consider how and when you want to share the news with the people you care about. And always be aware of any signs that indicate you need to rush to the doctor. These include heavy bleeding, severe abdominal pain, dizziness, and blurred vision.

The second trimester is often called the honeymoon phase of the pregnancy, as this is the time she'll feel best. She might even feel frisky during this stage. If this is the case, enjoy it. Your wife's tummy will grow fast, and people will start to notice the pregnancy. Your baby's kicks will become more robust, and soon your partner (and shortly after that, you) will feel these movements. There might be changes to her skin, including acne, stretch marks, dark marks on her face, and a dark line down her tummy. Now is a great time to look at taking birthing classes. During this trimester, you'll likely be able to find out the gender of your baby. Discuss with your wife if you want to know the gender and how you want to find out. Gender reveal parties are becoming very popular.

The third trimester will feel like a year, even though it's only three months long. Your wife will feel extremely uncomfortable. As this trimester progresses and the baby engages in the birth canal, she'll become even more uncomfortable. She'll experience pain at times due to her ligaments and muscles stretching. She might also start experiencing Braxton Hicks contractions. Read that again when it happens to your wife so you'll know whether your wife's experiencing these practice contractions or if it might be the start of true labor. Your wife will pee more than ever before. Stock up on two-ply toilet paper. Do this now if you still need to get the baby's room ready. Spoil her with a pedicure, help her to shave, and practice your go-to answers to trick questions such as "Do I look fat?"

When your wife's in the third trimester, start thinking about baby names if you haven't already decided on one. Decide if you want to choose a godparent for your child or who you'll appoint as your baby's guardian. Make sure they are stipulated in your will.

As the pregnancy progresses, pack the bags for the hospital. Remember to pack everything your partner, your baby, and you will need during labor and for at least three days after the baby has been born. When the labor starts, know when to go to the hospital. Unless your OB-GYN advises otherwise, remember the 5-1-1 rule: If her contractions are five minutes apart, each contraction lasts for one minute and has continued for one hour. Apart from contractions, other signs of labor to look out for include her mucus plug coming out (pinkish-brown Jell-O-like blob), having the urgent need for continuous bowel movements, and her water breaking.

When you're in the delivery room, never make a face showing any disgust, never call anything gross, and never tell her how long she has been in labor. Instead, try to help her in any way you can. Place a cold, damp cloth on her face if she's sweating. Allow her to squeeze the life out of your hand, don't tell her that her pain isn't "that bad," and please don't tell her when to push. Leave that to the trained professionals.

If there are complications, your OB-GYN will recommend delivering the baby via a C-section, and this isn't something you should fear. Know, however, that your wife's physical recovery will be longer, so be ready to help her in any way you can.

Once your baby has been born, be the gatekeeper. Only allow visitors once your partner and baby have settled into the maternity ward and all three of you are up for it. Remember to always make sure all visitors wash their hands and that they have no contagious diseases. If in doubt, don't let them in.

If your wife decides to breastfeed the baby, help her by getting snacks and ensuring she drinks enough fluids. Get involved in the feeds by burping the baby after every feed. Be there for your partner emotionally. Breastfeeding can be difficult and exhausting.

Before you know it, you'll take your baby home. Continue with your gatekeeper duties, but accept help when you and your wife need it, especially if someone offers to bring you a meal. Help out with chores around the house. Spend time with your baby by doing skin-to-skin contact. Take charge of bath time. And remember the importance of self-care, both for you and for your wife. You've both been through a lot, and caring for a newborn isn't an easy task.

Remember that dads don't babysit their children. They parent them. Be involved from the start by changing diapers and knowing how to handle and calm your baby. Spend quality time with your baby to bond. As soon as your baby becomes mobile, baby proof the house. Being the protector of your family is now part of your duties as a dad. Make sure you do everything you should to make your home as safe as possible for your tiny treasure.

Now that you have all the tools, go out there and use them. Be the dad you've always wanted to be. You'll rock this!

If you enjoyed reading this book and found the information helpful in preparation for your journey, please leave a review on Amazon.

To my new friend, cheers to being a Dad! I know you will rock.

- Alex

BIBLIOGRAPHY

Anderson, J. (2021, June 9). *5 sweet ways for dad to bond with baby*. Today's Parent. https://www.todaysparent.com/family/parenting/dad-struggling-to-bond-with-baby/

Babychakra. (2020, June 11). *10 things you must do to support your pregnant wife*. Swirlster. https://swirlster.ndtv.com/wellness-mother/10-things-you-must-do-to-support-your-pregnant-wife-2244348

Babylist. (2019, December 12). *Second trimester of pregnancy*. https://www.babylist.com/hello-baby/second-trimester

Barth, L. (2020, June 11). *Is pregnancy brain real?* Healthline. https://www.healthline.com/health/pregnancy/is-pregnancy-brain-real

Ben-Joseph, E. P. (2018). *Bringing your baby home*. Nemours Kids Health. https://kidshealth.org/en/parents/bringing-baby-home.html

Centers for Disease Control and Prevention. (2021, November 1). *Preterm birth*. https://www.cdc.gov/reproductivehealth/maternalinfanthealth/pretermbirth.htm

Coleman, P. A. (2020, May 5). *Building a birth plan: What expectant parents should include and consider*. Fatherly. https://www.fatherly.com/health-science/build-birth-plan-pregnancy-expecting

DiDonato, T. E. (2014, January 10). *5 reasons why couples who sweat together, stay together*. Psychology Today. https://www.psychologytoday.com/blog/meet-catch-and-keep/201401/5-reasons-why-couples-who-sweat-together-stay-together

Dragon, N. (2016, October 11). *Why pregnancy can make you have weird cravings*. Intermountain Healthcare. https://intermountainhealthcare.org/blogs/topics/   intermountain-moms/2016/10/why-pregnancy-can-make-you-have-weird-cravings/

Dubner, S. J. (2011, June 23). *It takes a village*. Freakonomics. https://freakonomics.com/2011/06/it-takes-a-village/

Gomstyn, A. (2022). *More than baby blues: Recognizing and recovering from postpartum depression*. Aetna. https://www.aetna.com/health-guide/ understanding-and-overcoming-postpartum-depression.html

Government of Victoria. (2012). *Childbirth - Pain relief options*. Better Health Channel. https://www.betterhealth.vic.gov.au/health/HealthyLiving/childbirth- pain-relief-options

Health America. (n.d.). *Mental health and the new father*. https://mhanational.org/mental-health-and-new-father

Healthdirect Australia. (2022). *Mental well-being during pregnancy*. Pregnancy Birth and Baby. https://www.pregnancybirthbaby.org.au/mental-wellbeing-during- pregnancy

Healthdirect Australia. (2020). *Third trimester*. Pregnancy Birth & Baby. https://www.pregnancybirthbaby.org.au/third-trimester

Hirsch, L. (2022). *Cesarean sections (C-sections)*. Nemours Kids Health. https://kidshealth.org/en/parents/c-sections.html

Kreidman, J. (2019, November 15). *Tips for new dads in the delivery room* [Video]. YouTube. https://www.youtube.com/watch?v=8G4e_NUkIeQ

Krieger, L. (2022, April 9). *First week at home with your newborn baby*. BabyCenter. https://www.babycenter.com/baby/newborn-baby/newborn-baby_10345806

Marcin, A. (2020, January 2). *How soon can you find out the sex of your baby?* Healthline. https://www.healthline.com/health/pregnancy/when-can-you-find- out-sex-of-baby

Mayo Clinic. (2018, September 1). *Postpartum depression*. https://www.mayoclinic.org/diseases-conditions/postpartum-depression/symptoms-causes/syc-20376617

Mayo Clinic. (2021, April 14). *Premature birth*. https://www.mayoclinic.org/diseases-conditions/premature-birth/symptoms-causes/syc-20376730

Mayo Clinic. (2022, March 9). *3rd-trimester pregnancy: What to expect.* https://www.mayoclinic.org/healthy-lifestyle/pregnancy-week-by-week/ in-depth/pregnancy/art-20046767

McKay, B. (2013, December 12). *New dad survival guide: The mindset.* The Art of Manliness. https://www.artofmanliness.com/people/fatherhood/new-dad- survival-guide-the-mindset/

McKay, B. (2021, May 30). *New dad survival guide: The skillset.* The Art of Manliness. https://www.artofmanliness.com/people/fatherhood/new-dad-survival-guide-the-skillset/

Merrell, C. (2022, March 24). *23 tips for new fathers.* Owlet. https://www.owletcare.com/blog/23-tips-on-becoming-a-father-for-the-first-time

National Health Service. (2020, December 1). *Signs that labour has begun.* https://www.nhs.uk/pregnancy/labour-and-birth/signs-of-labour/signs-that-labour-has-begun/

Procter & Gamble. (2021, November 22). *Hospital bag checklist—What to pack.* Pampers. https://www.pampers.com/en-us/pregnancy/giving-birth/article /what-to-pack-in-your-hospital-bag-go-bag-checklist

Rogers-Anderson, S. (n.d.). *10 expert tips to choosing a baby name.* The Tot. https://www.thetot.com/mama/10-expert-tips-for-choosing-a-baby-name/

Sandbox & Co. (n.d.). *Meaning and origin of Cameron.* Family Education. https://www.familyeducation.com/baby-names/name-meaning/cameronMental

Schools, D. (2018, September 24). *My 6 brutally honest fears about becoming a first-time dad.* Medium. https://daveschools.medium.com/my-6-brutally- honest-fears-about-becoming-a-first-time-dad-9464dcadc3af

Stewart, R. (2016, June 14). *Soon-to-be dads: How to help – And what not to say – During pregnancy.* UT Southwestern Medical

Center. https://utswmed.org/medblog/ fathers-guide-to-pregnancy/

Taylor, S. (2017, June 21). *The tricky task of choosing the right godparents for your baby.* Babyology. https://babyology.com.au/parenting/relationships/how-to- choose-godparents-for-your-baby/

Tiu, A. (2021a, April 11). *How to baby-proof your home 2021* [Video]. YouTube. https://www.youtube.com/watch?v=48BH4EuWTl4

Tiu, A. (2021b, May 25). *Sex after birth – Postpartum intimacy for new moms/dads* [Video]. YouTube. https://www.youtube.com/watch?v=JDIOz9jUGE4

Turner, A. (2020, June 23). *Delivery room tips for dads: 5 things not to do in labor* [Video]. YouTube. https://www.youtube.com/watch?v=VtjfS96qdnE

Watson, S. (2020a, July 16). *First trimester of pregnancy: What to expect.* WebMD. https://www.webmd.com/baby/guide/first-trimester-of-pregnancy

Watson, S. (2020b, August 25). *Second trimester of pregnancy.* WebMD. https://www.webmd.com/baby/guide/second-trimester-of-pregnancy

WebMD. (n.d.). *C-section: What can I expect?* https://www.webmd.com/baby/ what-happens-during-c-section#1

Welch, N. (2010, March 26). *A dad's point of view.* New Parent. https://newparent.com/mom/a-dads-point-of-view1/

Made in the USA
Monee, IL
06 May 2023